# HOMEOPATHY

## FOR

## COMMON AILMENTS

Robin Hayfield

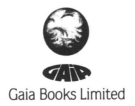

Gaia Books Limited

# A GAIA ORIGINAL

| | |
|---|---|
| Conceived by | Joss Pearson |
| Editorial | Eleanor Lines |
| | Janine Christley |
| | Fiona Trent |
| Design | Bridget Morley |
| Photography | Philip Dowell |
| Production | Susan Walby |
| Direction | Joss Pearson |
| | Patrick Nugent |

® This is a Registered Trade Mark
of Gaia Books Limited

First Published in the United Kingdom in 1993
by Gaia Books Limited

66 Charlotte Street        20 High Street
London W1P 1LR          Stroud, Glos GL5 1AS

Typeset by Tradespools Ltd,
Frome, Somerset, UK
Reproduction by Imago, Singapore
Printed by Mateu Cromo, Madrid, Spain

A catalogue record for this book is available from
The British Library

ISBN 1-85675-021-3

10 9 8 7 6 5 4 3 2

# HOMEOPATHY

— FOR —

## COMMON AILMENTS

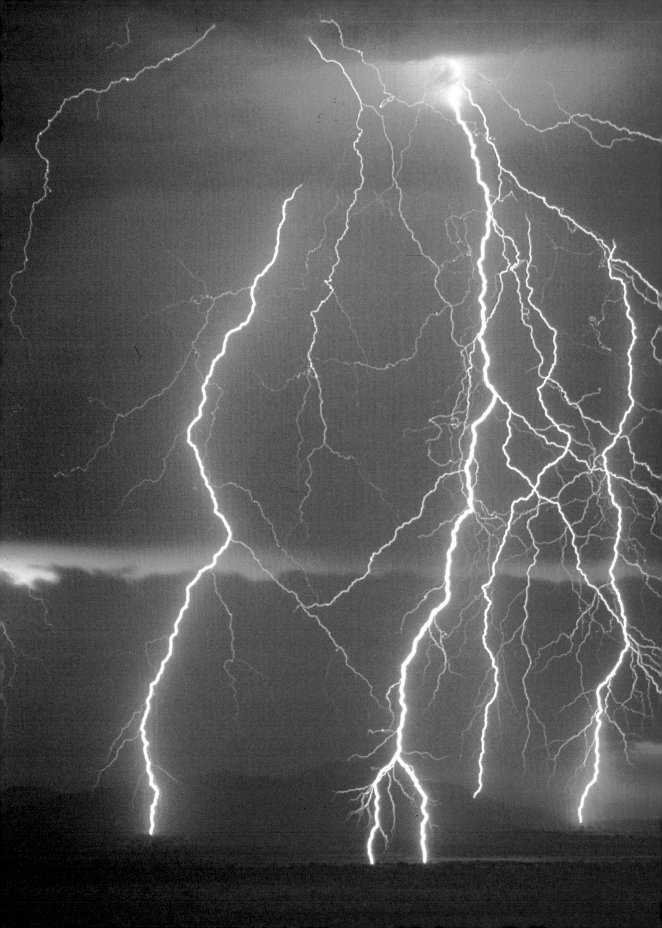

# How to use this book

*Homeopathy for Common Ailments* introduces homeopathy for everyone who wants gentle home treatment for everyday family health problems. Part One lists 37 common ailments. Under each ailment there is a description of several types of symptoms, both physical and mental. Match the patient's symptoms from the list and use the relevant remedy. Advice on dosage and when to seek medical advice is given on page 21.

Prescribing for Children follows the Common Ailments section. It describes the use of homeopathic remedies that are matched to personality types. As well as treating ailments, these remedies are useful as general tonics for children.

In Part Two there is a description of each remedy, giving its origin and uses. Use it to check the remedy you have chosen from Part One. The homeopathic remedy kit listed on page 92 gives the 20 remedies and five creams that are most commonly used. These will serve both as a first-aid kit and the basis of a collection for all your home treatment.

## The special language of homeopathy

Practitioners of homeopathy have a particular way of using language that may seem perplexing if you are exploring the subject for the first time. There are certain words, phrases, and language usages throughout this book, and in all other serious books on homeopathy, which should be explained to the newcomer:

## Constitutional type

For example: "the constitutional Arsenicum is very fastidious"

## Indication

For example: "Arnica is indicated" (if symptoms tell us that a certain remedy is likely to be beneficial)

## Keynote

For example: "sighing is a big Ignatia keynote" (a common body sign, habit, or signal that tells us that a remedy is likely to be of benefit to a sufferer)

## Remedies are used as adjectives

For example: "a Gelsemium influenza", or "in Belladonna cases"

## Remedies are described as "people" and their conditions

For example: "the pain of this remedy"

---

***Thunder and lightning*** *(frontispiece). People who respond well to the homeopathic remedy Phosphorous are usually spontaneous, uninhibited people who become very anxious during thunderstorms.*

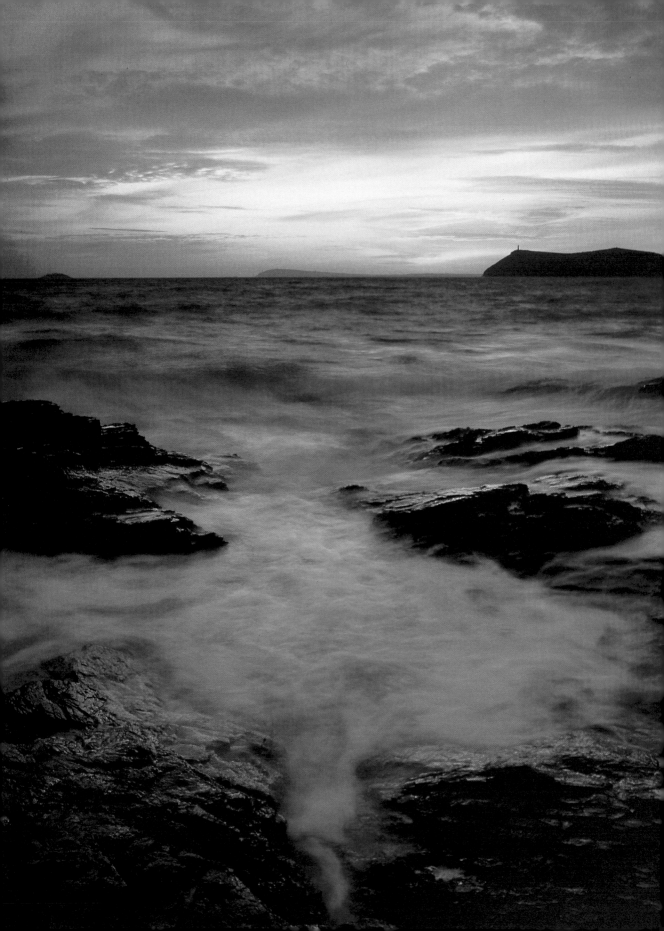

# CONTENTS

*The sea (facing page). Containing nearly 3% salt, sea water is the source of the remedy Natrum muriaticum. Symbolically the sea represents our deep, unconscious feelings. Nat mur types often conceal unresolved emotions such as grief and resentment beneath a calm exterior.*

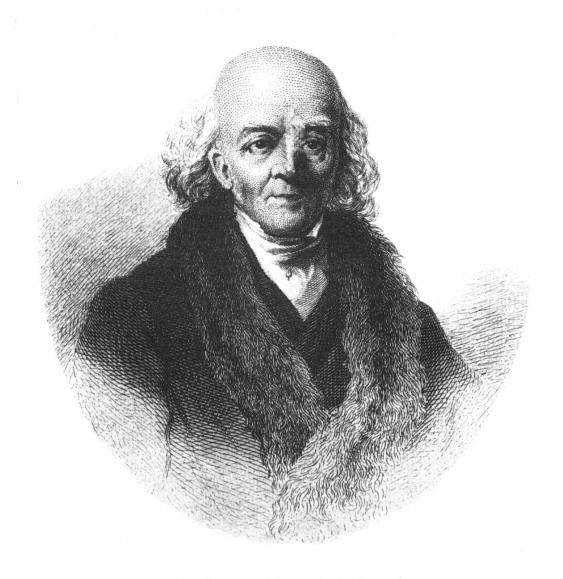

**Samuel Hahnemann**, *the founder of modern homeopathy.*

# Homeopathy –
## a sympathetic way of healing

One of the most gentle and sympathetic forms of healing, the practice of homeopathy, has been growing rapidly all over the world, particularly during the last decade. It has caught the imagination of many people who want to look at disease and healing in a different way.

Homeopathy is a thoughtful practice that respects the fact that every person is unique and individual. Homeopathic healing acts deeply on the organism, making lasting cures at all levels: physical, emotional, and mental. It is holistic, that is it treats the whole person, not just the disease. Many conventional doctors are not trained to look at the patient as a whole; they tend to treat each ailment separately and consequently the root cause is seldom found. The symptoms may disappear, but the disease is often merely suppressed, and recurs or surfaces again as another ailment, seemingly unconnected. Conventional medicine eases the discomfort of ailments with its painkillers, anti-inflammatory drugs, and anti-depressants, but side effects can be a major problem and a complete cure often remains out of reach.

This style of medicine, the dominant medicine in the West today, is known by homeopaths as the Way of Contraries, or healing through opposites. Disease is looked upon as an enemy, to be confronted and vanquished. The methods tend to be aggressive; our bodies are the battle grounds, with much talk of "fighting"; antibiotics and other drugs are employed as "magic bullets". Dangerous drugs and radioactive materials are used, along with a sophisticated array of knives and steel.

The word "homeopathy" is coined from ancient Greek; it means "similar suffering" – that like cures like. Homeopathy utilizes the natural Law of Similars, the principle that whatever can harm can also cure. Minute, safe doses are prescribed when someone exhibits the same symptoms as a larger dose of the same substance would have produced. Coffea is one example of this. Taken from coffee – a substance that stimulates the nervous system and causes sleeplessness if taken last thing at night – Coffea taken in tiny quantities does exactly the opposite. It has a soothing effect on the nerves and can help promote sleep.

## *The history of homeopathy*

For at least two thousand years philosophers interested in medicine have talked of these two different methods of healing. However, it was only two hundred years ago that the German physician and chemist, Samuel Hahnemann, finally formulated the laws and philosophy of homeopathy in a book called *The Organon*, which is still the bible of modern practitioners. During his long life (1755-1843) Hahnemann discovered many of the core remedies used today, which were sufficient to ensure that his medicine was thoroughly established. The whole practice of homeopathy is derived from his genius and experiments. Originally trained as an orthodox doctor, Hahnemann soon became disillusioned and appalled by the medical practices of the day. These included bloodletting in huge, and sometimes fatal, quantities, and the use of large doses of very poisonous drugs such as mercury, which caused untold damage. Such dangerous and unscientific methods persuaded Hahnemann to give up orthodox medicine. Instead he made a precarious living by writing, translating, and trying to find a more gentle way of healing. He was among the first to advocate the benefits of good hygiene and fresh air.

   In 1791 he translated an English article on the use of Peruvian bark, from which quinine is obtained to cure malaria. Struck by this, he started experimenting, testing small doses of the bark on himself. He noticed that he developed palpitations, became drowsy, and that his fingers and feet became quite cold. He noted symptoms of anxiety, with chilliness and tremblings, a marked thirst, and intense weakness. There was a numb, disagreeable sensation over the whole of his body. These symptoms occurred suddenly and regularly, lasting for about two or three hours. When he repeated the dose, they recurred. When he stopped taking the drug, the symptoms vanished and he recovered. Hahnemann

*Volcano (facing page). Sulphur is a product of volcanic eruptions and, like them, when used as a remedy it can bring disease to the surface.*

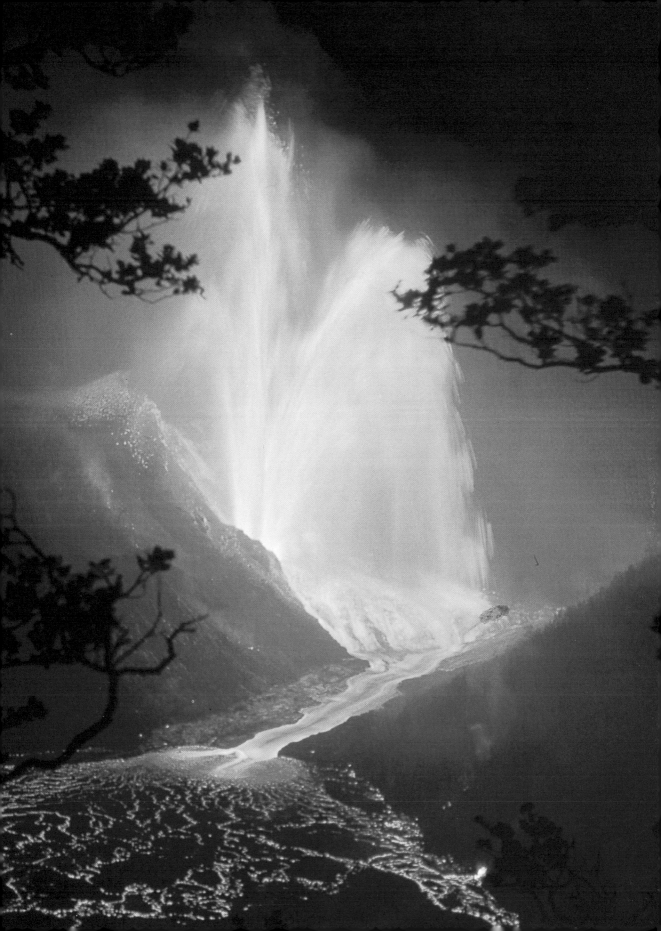

had produced in himself the symptoms of malaria, the very disease that Peruvian bark was supposed to cure.

Thus he started on the long road of rediscovery that like cures like, otherwise known as the Law of Similars. Hahnemann called this process of testing substances on healthy persons a "proving". It demonstrated that every remedy has imprinted in it a symptom picture. When the symptom picture that the remedy produces in a healthy person fits the characteristics of a patient, then a "similimum" is achieved and a cure will result. By the end of his life Hahnemann had scientifically "proved" over one hundred remedies on himself and on his colleagues. More than 2000 remedies have now been "proved", although a much smaller number are commonly used in practice. These are collected into the Materia Medica; an extremely detailed compilation of the symptoms of each remedy.

*Potentization through dilution and succussion*

Hahnemann was still concerned about the safety of even the small doses of the remedies he used, for some were prepared from very poisonous substances. He devised a method of dilution, with vigorous shaking, or "succussion", between each dilution that potentizes the remedy and seems to release and store huge reserves of curative energy.

Hahnemann invented a potency scale for the remedies according to the dilution. One part of the originial substance, or "mother tincture", diluted in 100 parts of alcohol or water is expressed as 1C. Diluted again one to 100 parts, the result, now one part in 10,000, is called 2C. One part in a million after three dilutions is 3C, and so on. C is the standard notation used for 100 and M is used for 1000. So, for example, 6C, the six hundredth potency, is the potency obtained when one part of the mother tincture is diluted in 100 parts of alcohol or water six times in succession. Correspondingly, 10M is the ten thousandth potency. Practitioners use the whole range, although seldom employ potencies above 10M. In this book the lower potencies – 6C or 30C – are ideal for home use. Potencies higher than 30C should only be prescribed by a qualified practitioner.

## The vital force

At a potency of around 9C a point is reached where not a single molecule of the original substance remains. No physical part of the remedy is left. The question then arises, how does it work? Hahnemann concluded that the remedy affected a part of the person that was non-material. This he called the "vital force" – the spirit that motivates the mind and uses the body for its physical expression.

The body is a self-adjusting mechanism that is usually perfectly capable of healing itself, unless there has been unnatural or persistent abuse. A parallel on a much bigger scale is Gaia, the vital force of the planet Earth, which regulates its temperature, oxygen and carbon dioxide levels, and biochemistry. In this way it maintains the best possible conditions for its own welfare and the life it supports.

However, like Gaia, the body sometimes sickens and needs help. Causes can be external, physical, and mental. Polluted water, earth, air, and additives in food are all external causes that our bodies are constantly struggling to assimilate. Physical causes include lack of sleep and exercise, addictions to tobacco, drugs, and alcohol, and bad eating habits with an over-consumption of sugar, meat, and fats. The emotional and mental stresses are less obvious, but probably more important, such as losing a loved one, fear of an employer or teacher, an unhappy marriage, or worries about one's children. Our ailments can result from our negative thinking and inappropriate emotional responses such as greed, jealousy, fear, excessive anger, resentment, and so on. A change of habit or environment may be needed to resolve the problem. The correct homeopathic remedy can not only cure the ailment but can help promote these changes and dig up the disease by the roots.

## The symptom picture

Symptoms are not regarded by homeopaths as ailments to be conquered at all costs. They are an expression of the distress in the vital force, and its attempt to make the necessary adjustments toward healing. The symptoms draw attention to the help that is needed. More often than not self-healing takes place as a result of rest, fresh air, and perhaps dietary adjustments. If we pay attention to it, the body tells us exactly what is needed for its recovery. But if not enough vitality is available, assistance is required from another source. The patient's symptoms will help to locate the curative remedy.

Ailments and symptoms are individual and peculiar to their owners. Each person expresses the symptoms of their ailment in different ways. One child's chickenpox may not be quite like another child's. My cough may be quite different from your cough. The most suitable remedy depends on the totality of symptoms, the evaluation of all the symptoms the patient is exhibiting, and for any one ailment you may consider a range of remedies. Always look for the remedy picture that fits most closely the picture of the symptoms.

### *Chronic and acute illness*

Acute illnesses generally tend to be short-lived and self-limiting. Examples include chickenpox, influenza, coughs, bites, and stings. Homeopathy eases the discomfort and speeds up healing. Some acute illnesses, however, such as meningitis, appendicitis, and pneumonia can be serious and need medical attention. All the acute illnesses dealt with in this book are suitable for home treatment, but read the caution on page 21 before commencing treatment.

Chronic diseases are longer-lasting, with deep-seated problems that are unlikely to clear up without treatment. These include skin problems, such as psoriasis, eczema, and acne, allergies, recurring asthma, recurrent colds, also any ailments that affect the vital organs of the body or the nervous system. The orthodox medical profession considers many such problems to be incurable, and can only alleviate the symptoms. Homeopathy however, can help curatively toward a cure in many of these chronic cases, but they are unsuitable for home treatment and must be referred to a qualified homeopathic practitioner.

*Aconite (facing page) is a very useful remedy for acute situations where there is extreme anxiety.*

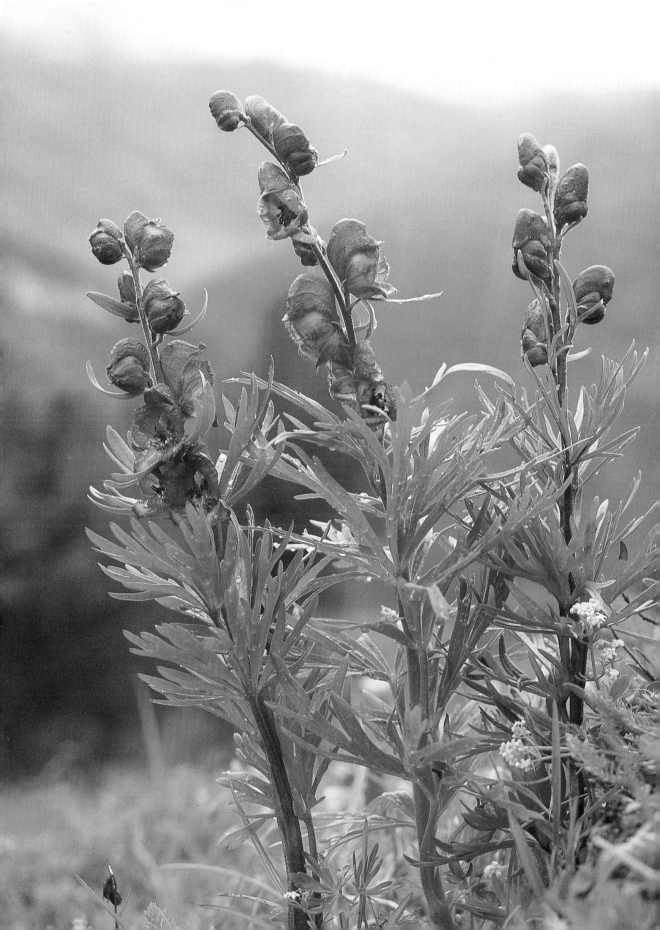

## The Laws of Cure

In the 19th century an American homeopath, Constantine Hering, observed that the body tries to push disease out to its extremities in its attempt to help itself. This protects the more essential organs, such as heart, liver, and lungs. For example, a dose of influenza after a period of overwork might, in fact, prove a blessing in disguise. The enforced rest eases the load on the nervous system, thus preventing something much more serious.

If, however, a superficial problem is suppressed, for example, by the use of a strong cortisone cream for a skin problem, then the disease may be driven inward and could result in asthma. The body is frustrated in its attempt to eradicate the disease through the periphery. Homeopaths always treat the deepest cause they can find. Only then can both the asthma and skin disease be resolved.

Hering's Laws of Cure describe not only the way that the body works to push disease out to the extremities. They also describe how the symptoms move from the top of the body to the lower regions. Symptoms are also cured in reverse order: the latest ailments disappearing first. In so doing, any disease that has been suppressed in the past may reappear briefly before disappearing completely. The best indication that you are improving is that you feel better in yourself. Then the cure is under way.

## Use at home

Homeopathy is a great comfort. With this book and some basic remedies you should be able to cope effectively with many of the common ailments and first-aid situations you will encounter. Some of the homeopathic remedies are specific to the ailment: use Arnica for bruises; Calendula for cuts and sores; Ledum for puncture wounds, and so on. These remedies often give extraordinarily quick results. When looking at the symptom picture try to see the person behind the disease; often aspects of their behaviour, or emotional characteristics, match a remedy picture. Is there a prominent thirst, or persistent food cravings; is the subject cold or hot and sweaty? Does s/he ask for fresh air or want the windows closed? What is the state of his/her breath? These are all helpful clues that individualize the case and can lead you to the correct remedy.

Don't worry if you initially give the wrong remedy, homeopathy is very safe and very forgiving. Try the next most likely remedy listed under the ailment. There are no side effects, though very occasionally the patient may feel a little worse before getting better. Except in first-aid and emergency cases, use homeopathy sparingly (see p. 21 for dosages). What you are trying to do is to help the body to heal itself; to give it a helping hand if things seem stuck. Imagine finding your car with a flat battery; give it a push start to get the car moving, then let the engine do the rest. Similarly, when you see that the healing process is in motion and the person feels better, stop repeating the remedy. Watch and wait. If the patient's symptoms recur, then repeat the remedy or give a different one to suit the new symptom picture. The healing process can be assisted by ensuring the patient eats plenty of fresh fruit and vegetables and whole grains, and takes a reasonable amount of exercise, with plenty of sleep.

Homeopathy can be used for almost all ailments, the main exception being mechanical problems, such as dislocation, many back problems, and cases of severe physical injury. Even so, homeopathy can ease the pain and speed up healing. Being a gentle form of healing, children tend to respond especially well, as do animals. Although it is based on scientific investigation, homeopathy is an art needing insight and feeling.

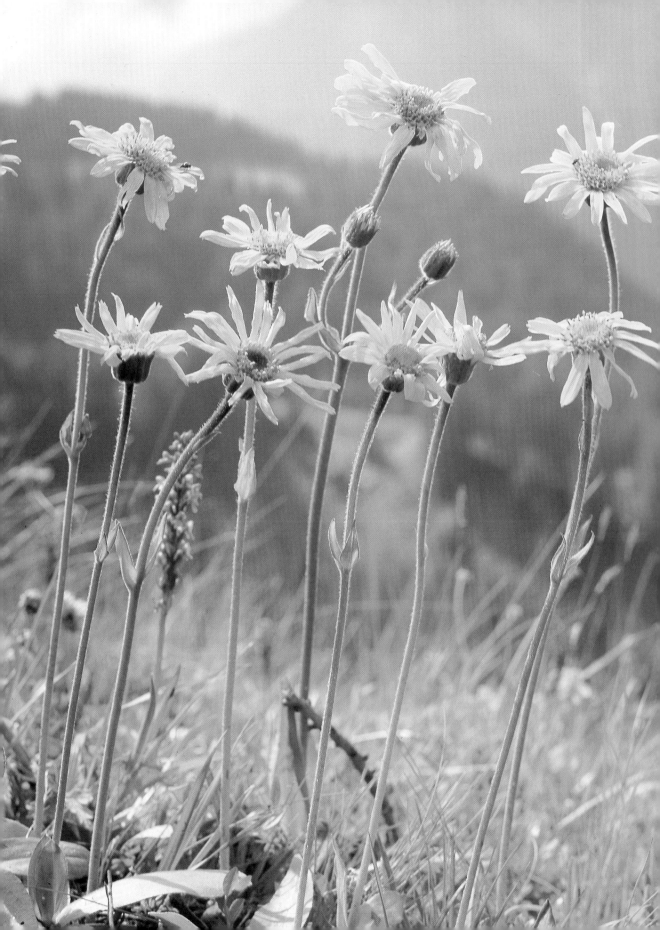

PART ONE
SECTION ONE

# THE COMMON AILMENTS

Anxiety and Anticipation
Asthma
Bites and Stings
Boils
Bruises
Burns
Chickenpox
Colds and Influenza
Colic
Coughs and Croup
Cuts and Injuries
Cystitis
Diarrhoea
Earache
Eye Injuries
Eye Strain
Eyes – Inflammation
Eyes – Styes
Fainting and Collapse

Fractures
Grief
Haemorrhoids
Hayfever
Indigestion
Measles
Mumps
Nausea and Vomiting
Nosebleeds
Shock
Sinusitis
Sore Throats and Tonsillitis
Sprains and Strains
Surgery and Dentists –
        before and after
Teething
Toothache
Travel Sickness
Whooping Cough

*Arnica (facing page) is an essential component of any first-aid kit since it is a wonderful remedy for bruises and accidents.*

# *Treating common ailments*

This chapter describes 37 common ailments that can be treated safely and easily by you at home, and offers a range of remedies for their treatment. Most of the ailments can be identified easily and few are likely to require diagnosis from an orthodox medical practitioner. The exceptions are mumps, measles, chickenpox, and whooping cough.

Firstly consult the list on page 19, then turn to the appropriate entry. Each ailment is presented in alphabetical order within the chapter. The general description of the symptoms will help to confirm your diagnosis and indicate the likely progress of the condition (though names of diseases are not of paramount importance to the homeopath). Several remedies are suggested; each one suiting a particular range of symptoms, both physical and emotional. The treatment will be more effective if the remedy covers your emotional and mental symptoms as well as the physical ones.

Read through all the remedy suggestions to see which of them matches the particular symptoms most closely. Once you have selected the remedy for the ailment, check it against the remedy entry in Part Two, the "Materia Medica" (see pp. 62-89), which gives a more detailed description of every remedy mentioned in the book. For information on dosages, see the facing page. If the treatment brings no improvement, find the remedy with the next closest match to the symptoms. See the facing page for instructions on handling and using the remedies.

The remedies suggested in this chapter should bring improvement or cure in most cases. Read the notes on each ailment carefully, and always consult a doctor where indicated. Do not treat skin diseases such as acne, eczema, or psoriasis. Homeopathic practitioners regard the skin as an organ of elimination for poisons from inside the body. To cure the skin without dealing with the problem that lies behind it merely suppresses the symptoms and can be counter-productive. Deep, chronic prescribing from a qualified homeopath is needed.

## Dosage

Use one remedy and one pill at a time. If there is no improvement after a day or so then try the next best remedy. In cases of emergency if there is no improvement after an hour change the remedy. As a general rule take one pill a day of the 30th potency, or one pill of the 6th potency three times a day. If the condition is really acute you can increase the frequency of the dosage to every few hours, or even hourly. Once you, or the sufferer, start to get better, stop taking the remedy. Having a clean tongue is helpful, so before you take the remedy, wait fifteen minutes before or after eating, or cleaning your teeth. Suck the remedy, don't just swallow it. Handle only the tablet you are taking. If you touch any others, or drop some, throw them away – don't put them back in the bottle.

## Caution

Serious illnesses and emergencies, of course, are beyond the scope of this book and need medical help. Warnings and cautions are included throughout the book indicating when this is necessary. Some conditions are obvious: no one should attempt to treat cancer, a stroke, asthma, or high blood pressure at home unaided. For persistent abdominal or chest pains, continuous bleeding, or any suspicious lumps, refer immediately to your doctor. For chronic diseases (any condition that does not clear up within a reasonable period after home treatment) consult a professional homeopath, who will prescribe constitutional or appropriate treatment. Use the golden rule: if in any doubt seek help.

# Anxiety and Anticipation

You will need the help of a homeopathic practitioner to treat chronic fears and anxieties, but there are a number of "one off" crises that you can usually treat yourself. These include worries and panics about taking exams, attending important interviews, meeting new people, flying, public speaking, taking a driving test, and many other similar problems. In extreme situations, use the Rescue Remedy (see p. 90), which you can use in addition to any other homeopathic remedy.

*Aconite*   You feel real terror and fright, and even fear of death. You "know" the plane is going to crash and nothing will save you! Try using Aconite before and after the event if you cannot shake off the nightmare feeling.

*Arg nit*   You feel anxiety rather than sheer terror; you simply cannot face the world and feel almost paralysed into inactivity. The anxiety can cause diarrhoea. Arg nit is a good claustrophobia remedy, so it may be useful if, for example, you are afraid of flying or travelling on underground trains.

*Arsenicum*   You cannot bear to be alone and feel very restless. You need constant reassurance that you will survive the ordeal. Midnight, or the hours after, can be a particularly bad time.

*Gelsemium*   You experience anticipatory fears, you feel weak and tired and your muscles will not obey your will. This remedy helps in situations that induce the "shakes and trembles".

*Phosphorus*   This remedy acts best if you are nervous and very sensitive; you feel much better in company. Twilight and shadows can cause you deep anxiety and sudden loud noises, such as a clap of thunder, tend to be very frightening.

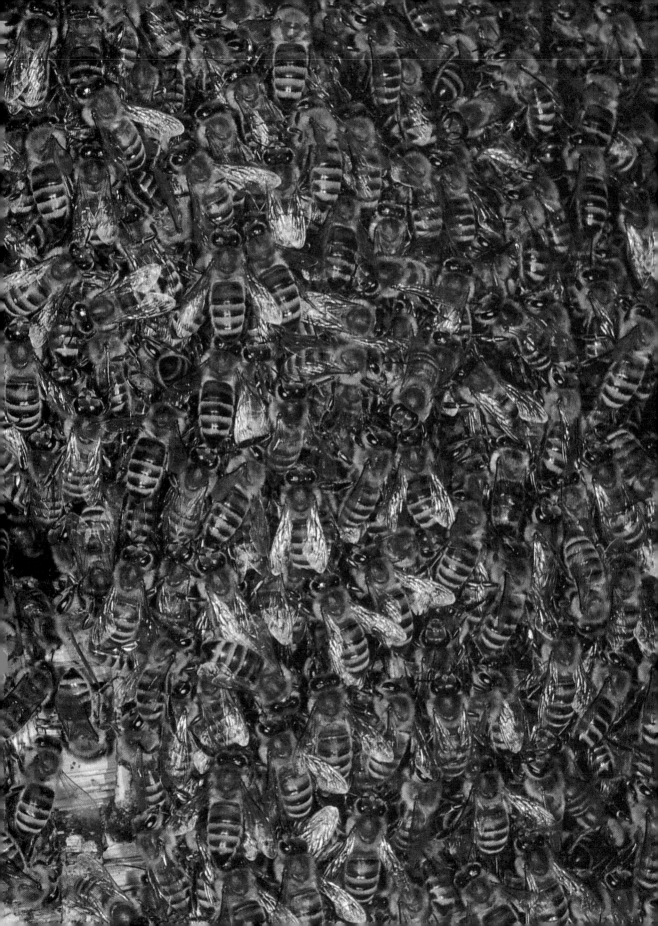

# Nausea and Vomiting

As in diarrhoea (see p. 32), vomiting is a natural process for the body to rid itself of something it does not want, in the quickest way possible. Nausea is usually the prior warning of this process, although it can mean other things too. Vomiting is commonly caused by an infection in the stomach or intestines that may be due to food poisoning or an infection of unknown origin. If the vomiting and nausea clear up reasonably quickly and you are feeling better then you do not need to take any homeopathic medicines. However, if it is persistent and you feel your body is not coping well, then choose one of the following remedies. Some of the remedies in the diarrhoea section (see p. 32) help ease vomiting as well.

*Arsenicum* This is frequently the first remedy to consider in acute ailments of the gastrointestinal tract. Use it when diarrhoea and stomach pains accompany violent vomiting. Other symptoms include weakness and exhaustion, chilliness, and restlessness. You may want to take sips of cold water, which you then vomit straight up again. Take Arsenicum on holiday with you, especially where you are doubtful about the level of hygiene in the local food and water.

*Bryonia* If you have stomach pains you want to lie quite still on the side that hurts and to be left completely alone. In spite of the vomiting, you are very thirsty and want lots of cold water.

*Colocynthis* The vomiting is accompanied by the most unbearable stomach pains, which come in spasms like colic. The only thing that seems to ease the agony is doubling up or pressing the painful part very hard.

*Ipecac* Vomiting does not seem to help the extreme nausea and you feel just as bad afterwards. Your tongue remains clean and does not become coated. Overeating may be the cause of the symptoms.

*Nux vomica* You may feel a great urge to vomit, but despite the nausea you fail to bring much up. The cause may be overeating or too much rich food. It is often the remedy for the business person who eats too much, works too hard, and takes too little exercise. The undigested food feels like a heavy load in the stomach. You may feel noticeably irritable and chilly.

*Phosphorus* The symptoms are similar to those of Arsenicum (see above) and you should use it if Arsenicum does not work. A peculiarity of this remedy is that you want cold drinks, which are vomited up as soon as the liquid is warmed in the stomach. Sometimes you may have an empty hollow feeling in the stomach.

*Apis mellifica* (previous page), whose source is the honey bee, has many uses, including first aid for bites and stings.

## Nosebleeds

Injury can cause nosebleeds, but some people are prone to them for no apparent reason. Usually they stop of their own accord, but if they do not, try one of the following remedies:

*Arnica*  Use Arnica to help reabsorb the blood of nosebleeds resulting from an injury.

*Phosphorus*  This remedy is a good all-purpose haemorrhage remedy useful for persistent nosebleeds that pour without warning or apparent reason.

## Shock

In medical terms, shock is produced by a sudden fall in the amount of circulating blood, which leads to a lack of oxygen in the tissues and organs. The symptoms include a weak pulse, shallow breathing, cold, pale skin, fainting, and anxiety. The causes of shock cover the whole range of physical and emotional trauma.

If shock follows a severe accident, or if the reason seems incomprehensible, seek medical help immediately. Meanwhile keep the sufferer warm and loosen any tight clothing. Do not move him or her if there is a serious injury or s/he is unconscious. Otherwise move the head to a position lower than the body so that the blood drains back to the head. Give the Rescue Remedy every few minutes (see p. 90). A few drops on the lips will do – it can be a real life-saver.

*Aconite*  This is the great remedy for terror and fear of death. It is particularly useful if you take it retrospectively to help you recover from a past event or experience that has left you with deep physical or emotional scars.

*Arnica*  This wonderful medicine is the number one remedy for shock, as well as for bruising. In an accident, therefore, it serves a double purpose. In emergencies repeat the dose every few minutes in conjunction with Rescue Remedy. For an unconscious person, who must not take anything by mouth, place a tiny bit of the crushed pill on the lips.

## Sinusitis

Sinuses are small cavities in the bones around the eyes and above the nose. In sinusitis, the membranes inside the cavities become swollen and inflamed and the symptoms are a blocked nose, discharge, and sometimes pain and fever in more severe cases. Colds or allergies may begin the inflammation. The remedies that help are usually the common cold remedies. See the section on Colds and Influenza (p. 29).

# Sore Throats and Tonsillitis

Sore throats can result from both viral or bacterial infection, catarrh, or dryness of the membranes. Usually the symptoms clear fairly quickly without treatment, although the bacterial infection known as "strep throat" (streptococcus) can be more persistent and may require medical help.

Tonsillitis is an inflammation of the tonsils, the two little organs situated at the back of the throat, which can become painfully swollen from infection. Chronic sore throats or persistent tonsillitis require constitutional homeopathic treatment. The following remedies should cover most acute cases:

*Aconite* The symptoms appear suddenly, often after getting a chill. Your throat feels hot and dry. It is difficult to swallow, which may be frustrating, as you are sometimes very thirsty. The pain usually starts in the middle of the night or is worse at that time.

*Apis* Redness, puffiness, and stinging are the prominent symptoms in Apis throats. Cool drinks help, although you are not usually thirsty.

*Belladonna* As in Aconite, there is a sudden onset of symptoms, but with little or no thirst. The temperature is high, your face is red, and your pupils dilated. The tonsils will appear bright red and the pain is best described as a throbbing one.

*Hepar sulph* The feeling of a fish bone sticking in the throat describes the pain of this remedy. The throat is very sore and you may cough up green mucus. You feel very bad tempered and cannot bear to be even slightly cold.

*Lachesis* These throats are usually distinctive because swallowing solids is less painful than swallowing liquids. There is a feeling of a lump or swelling in the throat. The pain is most often left-sided or begins on the left and moves to the right and it may extend to the ear. You cannot bear any constriction around your throat or chest area.

*Lycopodium* These throats are right-sided, or worse on the right, or move from right to left. Warm drinks help and you may feel worse in the late afternoon or early evening.

*Mercurius* Your breath may smell and you may have profuse yellow, slimy saliva. Your throat feels raw and your tongue looks swollen and flabby. You are usually sweaty and rather thirsty.

*Phytolacca* Your throat looks dark or bluish-red inside. The pain is especially bad on swallowing and feels like a hot lump in the throat. The rest of your body may ache.

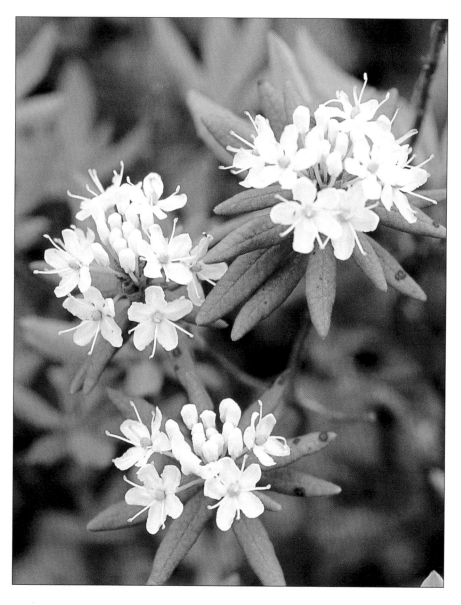

***Ledum****. The remedy derived from this shrub is a notable first-aid treatment for puncture wounds. Injuries feel cold, yet strangely feel better for cold compresses rather than hot ones.*

## Sprains and Strains

Sprains and strains are injuries to the connecting tissues that surround the joints. These are the ligaments, which connect bone to bone and tendons, which connect muscle to bone. A sprain is a partially torn ligament or tendon; a strain is when the tissue has been overstretched.

*Arnica*  It is a good idea to first use Arnica cream as an external application to ease the bruising and soreness. If you use it in this way, you can combine it with another internal remedy, where applicable.

*Bryonia*  Whenever the pain feels worse from the slightest movement, use Bryonia. The pain may be so bad that the only thing that helps is to hold the injured part very tightly. For this reason, Bryonia is particularly useful for the pain of dislocation as well as for sprains.

*Ledum*  Injuries that require Ledum look purple and puffy and feel cold. Cold compresses help.

*Rhus tox*  This remedy is probably the most commonly used medicine for sprains. In classic cases the pain is worse initially, but eases if you exercise the joint a little bit. Warmth, hot baths, and rubbing should also help, in addition to rest and a firm bandage. Rhus tox can be helpful for any type of muscle strain.

*Ruta*  This remedy has an affinity with the periosteum, the membrane covering the bone surface. Use it when the bones themselves feel bruised. It is a good tennis elbow remedy. Try Ruta if Rhus tox does not work.

## Sunburn – see Burns (p.28)

## Surgery and Dentist – before and after

Homeopathy can help after surgery and dental treatment in two ways. For worry and anticipation see the section Anxiety and Anticipation on page 22. Treatment can also help with the accompanying shock and injury, which sometimes feels as painful as the operation itself.

*Arnica*  This rememdy is almost always the first remedy to think of for the shock and bruising that are virtually inevitable after major dental work or surgical operations. Take Arnica 30C immediately afterwards, and then as you feel necessary. If you are particularly frightened then take the remedy before treatment as well.

*Calendula*  Use Calendula for open cuts and wounds; externally as a cream or diluted tincture directly to the area around the incision.

*Hypericum*  Consider using Hypericum if you have injuries to the nerves. The pain characteristically shoots along the nerve tracks. You can use Hypericum instead of Arnica, or if Arnica does not work, after operations to such areas as the nose, fingers, toes, eyes, ears, or gums.

*Phosphorus* This is a very useful remedy. Phosphorus will stop excessive bleeding after an operation, such as a tooth extraction, in a sensitive person. Also use it to alleviate that post-anaesthetic "spaced-out" feeling.

*Staphysagria* The emotional picture of Staphysagria includes the feeling of an unwelcome invasion of your private space. Consider using it in post-operative cases where you feel you have been insensitively handled, humiliated, or violated during painfully rough dentistry, or childbirth involving an episiotomy or forceps delivery. Also consider Staphysagria when the pain or scars are slow to heal in addition to the emotional indignation you feel.

## Teething

Most parents have experienced the frustration of watching the pain and discomfort of their babies as the first teeth come through. Homeopathy can usually help to ease the pain.

*Chamomilla* This remedy usually eases teething pain. The baby is cross, perhaps throwing his or her toys across the room, and wants to be carried or rocked gently. One cheek may be red and the other pale.

*Pulsatilla* Emotionally, Pulsatilla children are the opposite of the bad-tempered Chamomilla ones. When teething, Pulsatilla children will be whingeing and clingy. Cool, fresh air helps them.

## Toothache

The agonizing pain of toothache always seems to start at weekends, or when you are on holiday and there are no dentists to be found. The pain is usually caused by decay, gum disease, or an abscess. In the case of an abscess, pus is trapped in a cavity. You can relieve the pressure that this creates by applying hot compresses and washing your mouth out continually with warm salt water. The release of pus eases the pain. Nonetheless, you should see a dentist.

*Belladonna* These abscesses tend to come up very quickly and you should use Belladonna early on in their development. The area looks red, hot, and swollen, your mouth feels dry and the tooth throbs painfully.

*Mercurius* Your gums feel very sore and painful and will probably bleed. The pain is worse at night and it feels as though a lot of pus is present. You are thirsty, have more saliva than usual, and your breath smells bad.

*Hepar sulph* The pain feels like sharp splinters and is very sensitive to touch and to cold air. An abscess needing this remedy will be very septic, slow to heal, and may ooze thick, yellow, foul-smelling pus. You will feel cold, irritable, and very bad tempered.

*Silica* This is a good remedy to try when the abscess will not come to a head or is slow to heal. The onset is also slow. Silica teeth are often not in very good condition and you may already have sepsis, caries, and discolouring.

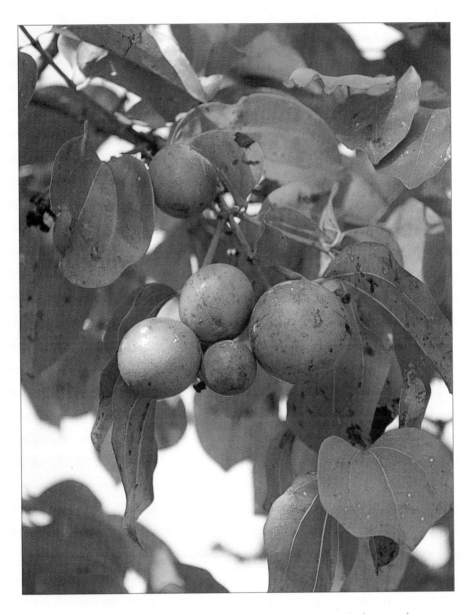

***Nux vomica****. The seeds of the Poison Nut Tree produce a remedy that eases the discomfort of indigestion. It has many other uses too and is a useful first-aid remedy.*

## Travel Sickness

The symptoms of motion sickness are nausea, dizziness, and vomiting, which may be brought on by car, boat, and aeroplane travel; car sickness affects young children more than adults, while seasickness can occur at any age.

*Cocculus*  This remedy covers all the symptoms so try it first. You desperately want to lie down and food, or even the thought of food, can bring on a feeling of nausea.

*Tabacum*  You experience extreme nausea and violent vomiting from the slightest motion. You look very pale, sweat profusely, and feel better in cool, fresh air.

## Whooping cough

Whooping cough is an acute bacterial infection of the respiratory tract. It usually affects young children, but is only really dangerous in children under a year old. The symptoms normally start with a slight fever and can be confused with the common cold. The famous "whoop" does not happen until at least a week later, when the child starts to try and cough up the thick mucus trapped in the lungs. The "whoop" is the sound that is made in the attempt to replace the expelled air. The coughing fits can last weeks, and very occasionally, months, and is very distressing for both child and parents. However, it sounds more alarming than in fact it is. You will probably feel happier in seeking medical help, and for a very tiny child it is vital that you should. In the early stages, before the cough starts, consult the Colds and Influenza section (see p. 29) for a suitable remedy. Once the "whoop" starts, then the following remedies apply. See also the Coughs and Croup section (p. 30).

*Bryonia*  The cough is dry, hard, and very painful. It is worse for eating and drinking, despite a great thirst. The slightest movement exacerbates the cough, so the child may hold his or her chest very tightly during coughing. The membranes surrounding the lungs are very dry; this lack of lubrication causes the pain.

*Coccus cacti*  Outbursts of the violent, tickling cough can end in vomiting, with profuse, ropey mucus hanging from the mouth. Cold drinks help. Lying in a warm bed exacerbates the coughing fits.

*Drosera*  The incessant paroxyms happen very quickly one after the other and sound like a deep barking. The cough seems to come from the abdomen, and the child may hold his or her sides. The choking cough may result in retching and vomiting. Drosera symptoms are worse for lying down. The worst time is after midnight.

*Ipecac*  This remedy's conditions feature prominent nausea and vomiting of mucus, which is sometimes bloody. The child has a rattly chest, feels suffocated, and stiffens up.

# PART ONE
# SECTION TWO

# *Prescribing for children*

The remedies for common ailments give in Section One (see pp. 20-51) apply equally to adults and to children. But there exists another method of home prescribing: the constitutional remedy. This type of remedy has a broad symptom picture, which can affect the whole nature or constitution. It may match the personality of people of all ages, but in children we can see the correlations more easily. The following six constitutional remedies are by no means comprehensive, but they are probably the most common. People often display a mixture of remedy types, but one may tend to dominate.

Read and study these remedy pictures. If you can see one that fits your child, you have at your disposal another method of prescribing. The constitutional remedy acts as a general tonic. It may not matter very much what the child is suffering from; give the constitutional remedy and the child may simply rise above the disease.

Think of using this method particularly in chronic states – for the child who often suffers from earache, or who never seems able to shake off a cold properly, and so on. Learn to see the child in a different, holistic, way: if your rumbustious child represents the Sulphur type, give him or her a dose of Sulphur; if your baby is unusually needy s/he should respond to Pulsatilla.

### *DOSAGE*
While the child is feeling unwell, give one 30C pill daily until the child starts feeling better. Otherwise give occasionally as a general tonic if the child seems a bit under the weather.

## *CALCAREA CARBONICA*

Calcarea children like to set their own pace and are unhappy if people force them to do things that they are not prepared for. Their favourite speed is slow, both mentally and physically; they are just as intelligent as other types, but they need time to learn new things, to assimilate and categorize the outside world. Such children may appear to be obstinate and inflexible, but they need to understand what is going on before they act. Often late developers, they may be slow to teethe; and their fontanelles close more slowly than other children's. They walk late, talk late, and at school they tend to be plodders rather than the class stars. Independent and serious children, they enjoy playing by themselves. Sensitive to ridicule, they will avoid situations where their slowness and native caution may show them up. Despite their introverted, easy-going nature, they are capable of temper tantrums if they are pushed beyond what they feel is their natural limit.

These children need to feel safe: they are not adventurous and do not like heights. They may be scared of the dark and shadows, they fear ghosts and scary monsters on the television, and may become very nervous if mice or spiders cross their path. Dogs may also cause them problems. Nightmares cause them to wake up screaming and they often worry about the future; they need to be reassured that calamities will not befall them, and why not. Sometimes they are interested in the supernatural, and ask a lot of questions about God at a very young age.

Calcarea carbonica children love stodgy food – bread, pasta, and all carbohydrates, and have a marked craving for eggs, especially soft-boiled ones. Babies will often want to eat chalk or earth in the garden. They usually dislike meat, and milk often disagrees with them. They tend to be constipated and can often go for days without a bowel movement, but strangely it does not seem to cause them discomfort. Physically they are usually quite plump and rather sweaty, especially on the hands and head; at night you may find damp patches on the pillow. Their ankles may be weak and prone to strains. They feel the cold in their head and so like to have it covered. These children are prone to colds, coughs, earache, sore throats, and tonsillitis; these ailments are caused or exacerbated by the cold and damp. They generally feel much better in the warmth. They may suffer from fevers with high temperatures, which may require Belladonna as an acute remedy (see p.69).

CONSTITUTIONAL REMEDY II

## *LYCOPODIUM*

Lycopodium children have one major problem: lack of self-confidence, but you would not always guess it. Some of them disguise it with a cover-up act and can be fault-finding, bossy, and dictatorial, playing a power game with their parents and with other children. But on the other hand they appear to be timid and nervous with strangers and need the comforting presence of someone to turn to for reassurance. These children can suffer dreadfully from the worries of anticipation: the fear of exams, of speaking in front of the class, or being seen to be a failure. They take themselves seriously and hate being made to look a fool. They crave the good opinion of others in order to boost an ego that is not always very well defined. They cry after being reprimanded and are therefore frightened of making mistakes, such is their sensitivity. Life can be filled with compromise, as decisiveness is not their strong point. Unsure of themselves, there can be a marked fear of fresh challenges or meeting new people. They fear the dark, ghosts, and large animals and they may need a night light or someone to sleep with when they are very young.

Physically these children are often thinner than average, with a large head in proportion to their body. They are slow to smile until they feel safe and even babies appear to wear a wrinkly frown. They feel the cold, although they like their head to be cool. The late afternoon and early evening are bad times for Lycopodium children, and they are particularly cross when they wake up or when they feel hungry. The stomach is usually a weak point in Lycopodium children. Fear and anxiety go straight there, so they suffer from wind and constipation. They should avoid foods that aggravate their wind, such as cabbage, beans, and onions. They often have a huge appetite, but conversely, they sometimes feel full up after having eaten only a few mouthfuls. They love sweets and choose warm food and drinks.

These children are subject to most childhood ailments, but especially earache, and colds and coughs, which may move down to the chest, causing bronchitis. Symptoms tend to begin on the right side of the body and move to the left, or are worse on the right side. Eczema sometimes affects the head, especially behind the ears. A child who has repeated colds and infections, and whose general personality and physical characteristics fit in with the above description will benefit from Lycopodium.

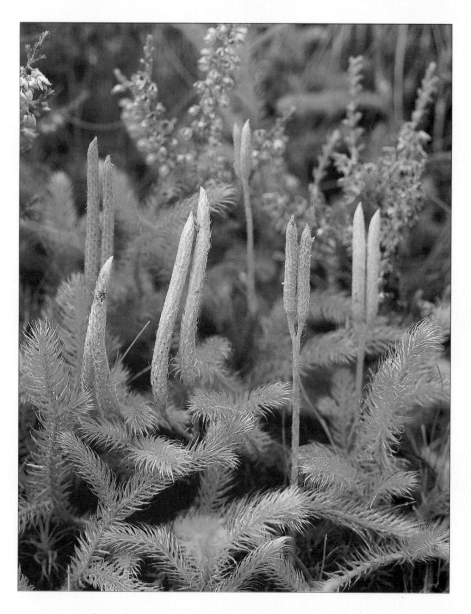

**Lycopodium** (foreground). The spores of this primitive and strange-looking plant
are the source of one of the most important remedies in the whole Materia Medica.
Lycopodium affects the digestive system and is also a major constitutional remedy
where the personality fits the symptom picture.

CONSTITUTIONAL REMEDY III

# *NATRUM MURIATICUM*

Nat mur children are emotionally extremely sensitive. They are usually reserved, introverted, and feel things very deeply, finding it difficult to share or communicate their problems. Very easily hurt, and knowing what pain is like, they are sensitive about hurting others. Being told off is a terrible ordeal, so they behave well to avoid it. When they cry, they prefer to do so alone in their room, maybe playing sad music as consolation, and to release their locked-up feelings. They are well organized and are often perfectionists, keeping themselves and their rooms neat and tidy.

Self-contained and independent by nature, they enjoy being alone. They worry about what people think of them and fear being the centre of attention, so parties are not much fun for them. Being very self-conscious, they hate being seen to make mistakes. Easily embarrassed, they dislike praise or being comforted, except by a very "safe" person.

Often they appear to be wise and reponsible beyond their years and such children can be very hard on themselves and filled with guilt and sadness. Even their parents may never be aware of their fears. Nor might you ever guess that inner resentment can be a big issue. These children have long memories and are often slow to forgive; many of their problems result from their locked-up emotions. Nat mur is one of the major grief remedies – children who need it may often have some emotional trauma in their backgrounds, such as the divorce of their parents, or the loss of a friend or pet. This unexpected sadness can make them physically ill. They are frightened of anything that is out of their control – burglars, spiders, or the thought that their parents might die.

These children dislike a stuffy atmosphere or being outside in the hot sun, which can give them hammering headaches. They often crave salt and salty foods, and their ailments usually worsen in the sea air, though occasionally this can make them feel better. Nat mur children may suffer allergies, such as hayfever, or be allergic to certain foods. They tend to dislike fatty or slimy foods. Although they eat well, they find it hard to put on weight. They suffer from cold sores around their lips, and when they have a cold the discharge is thin and clear, and more whitish than the normal green-yellow discharge. Nat mur can help them release their spontaneity and make them well.

CONSTITUTIONAL REMEDY IV

## *PHOSPHORUS*

Everyone seems to love Phosphorus children. They are a delight; warm-hearted, sympathetic, and affectionate, they attract others like a magnet, which suits them very well, for they love company. It is particularly important that someone who loves them is near by or, better still, holding them when they are ill.

They are naturally extrovert children, full of spontaneity and curiosity, tending to be restless and always into new things. In fact, they can easily make themselves sick through sheer excitement or through the overplay of a very vivid imagination. They give out a lot and need a lot of attention in return, but such is their good nature and playfulness that nobody minds too much. Phosphorus children are seldom shy and on the occasions that they are, it proves very endearing and is easily overcome if they are given praise or affection.

If Phosphorus children have a fault it is that they are not always very focused and are easily distracted from the matter in hand. They can be nervous and they are sometimes highly strung. Thunderstorms really frighten them and they are afraid of the dark and shadows at twilight. They may like a parent to see them off to sleep in case there is a ghost in the room, though a night light may comfort them. Another worry may be that something dreadful will happen to their parents or the people they care for.

Physically they are delicate-looking children, likely to be tall and thin, with good skin and long eyelashes. They tend to be thirsty and love cold drinks. They frequently adore ice cream (though what child doesn't?) and may be fond of spicy foods. They sometimes feel faint if their blood sugar level falls too low, so it is best not to let them miss meals. The stomach can be a weak point and a peculiarity is that sometimes, when they are ill they vomit cold food and drink as soon as it has warmed up inside. They have loose stools and constipation is rare. Nosebleeds can be a problem, and they are prone to sore throats and may also become hoarse. Colds tend to go straight to the chest (another weak area); laryngitis can quickly turn to bronchitis, and they will complain of tightness and heaviness.

You will always know when a Phosphorus child is sick as they are very open and expressive about their problems. They feel better for being consoled and cuddled and are living proof that, combined with a few pills of Phosphorus, love is much the best remedy.

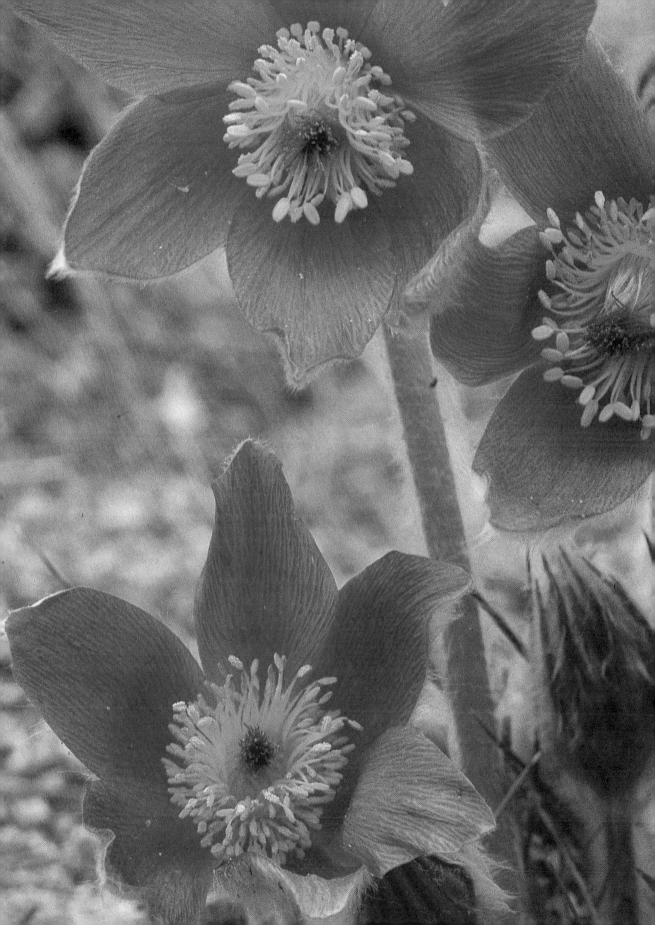

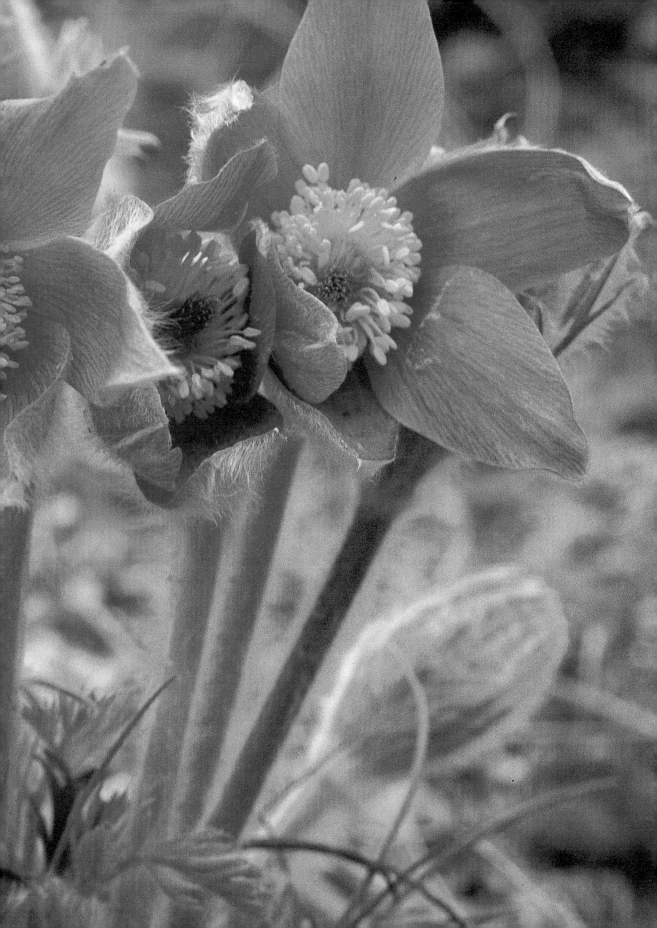

CONSTITUTIONAL REMEDY V

## *PULSATILLA*

Fear of abandonment is the dominating issue for Pulsatilla children. They are mild, gentle souls, rather timid and very eager to please. This ensures approval from their parents or their friends so that they are not rejected.

They tend to be weepy children under stress with a clingy, fearful nature, keeping close to their parents in unfamiliar situations. They are very "good" children, doing what they are told; very sensitive to reprimand, they break down easily if told off. Although they have an affectionate and loving nature, there is also a jealous and touchy side to their personality. This can appear when they feel pushed to the sidelines by a brother or sister who seems to be getting all the attention. Because they are ultra-sensitive, you can sometimes trace their ailments back to a particular sad event, such as their best friend moving to a new school.

Their moods are very up and down – crying one moment and laughing the next. This is of course true of most tiny children, but the changeable Pulsatilla nature carries on like this long after you feel they should have grown out of it. They are easily consoled by affection and sympathy and, best of all, by being allowed into their parents' bed at night.

Pulsatilla children are warm-blooded and feel best out in the fresh air. They are not thirsty children and when they do drink they prefer it cool. Rich, fatty foods disagree with them and may cause diarrhoea and vomiting.

They are very indecisive children – it is a real problem getting them to make up their mind about anything. When they are ill, their symptoms – like their nature – are changeable. Pains shift from one area to another – one moment it is their chest, the next it is their stomach. They are prone to earache, colds that move to their chest, and often they have a blocked nose, full of yellow-green mucus. They can also be susceptible to recurring styes.

All ailments respond well to sympathy, a good cry, cold compresses, and fresh air, as well as the remedy Pulsatilla.

*Pulsatilla (previous page). The remedy derived from the Pasque or Windflower is a major polycrest or remedy with many uses, and is a cure for numerous ailments.*

CONSTITUTIONAL REMEDY VI

## *SULPHUR*

Sulphur children stand out in a crowd. Full of energy and curiosity they are natural leaders with a well-developed sense of self. Naturally quick and intelligent they assimilate new information fast and are not afraid to put it to practical use. There is another Sulphur type who is quieter, but equally intelligent and curious and with the annoying habit of "knowing it all". Both types are always asking questions and their persistence sometimes drives their parents to utter exasperation. Sulphur types are naturally self-confident and somewhat opinionated. Rather egocentric they do not usually care what others think of them and so easily upset those with more sensitive feelings. They often believe that rules are for breaking and are seldom frightened of the consequences.

They are messy children – their rooms defy description and they are not particular about their appearance. Lazy by nature, and the world's greatest procrastinators, they would rather slouch in a chair than stand. Despite their strong, restless personality, Sulphur children are quite good-natured and enjoy giving a helping hand, especially when they can demonstrate how much better they are than anyone else.

Physically they are usually big and strong for their age, although the quieter types may be thinner. They may be quite red-faced and can be prone to skin problems such as eczema, which itches and burns, especially after a bath. Bathing in any case is not their strong point and they can look quite unwashed. When they are small, they are the children you see with runny noses, sweaty heads, red eyes and ears, and not always very "civilized" habits. They do not feel the cold and may stick their feet out of bed at night to cool them off. Their low time is about 11am, when they may become very hungry. They normally like sweet things and strong-flavoured foods. They are quite thirsty children, but they may be allergic to milk.

As one might imagine, not much frightens Sulphur children, although they may be scared of heights. They are relatively strong constitutionally, but when they are ill they lose all their natural exuberance and become quite dull and lethargic. Any ailment can trouble them, and they are rather susceptible to skin problems. Parents should therefore devote extra time to keeping these children clean and hygienic, which can be an uphill struggle.

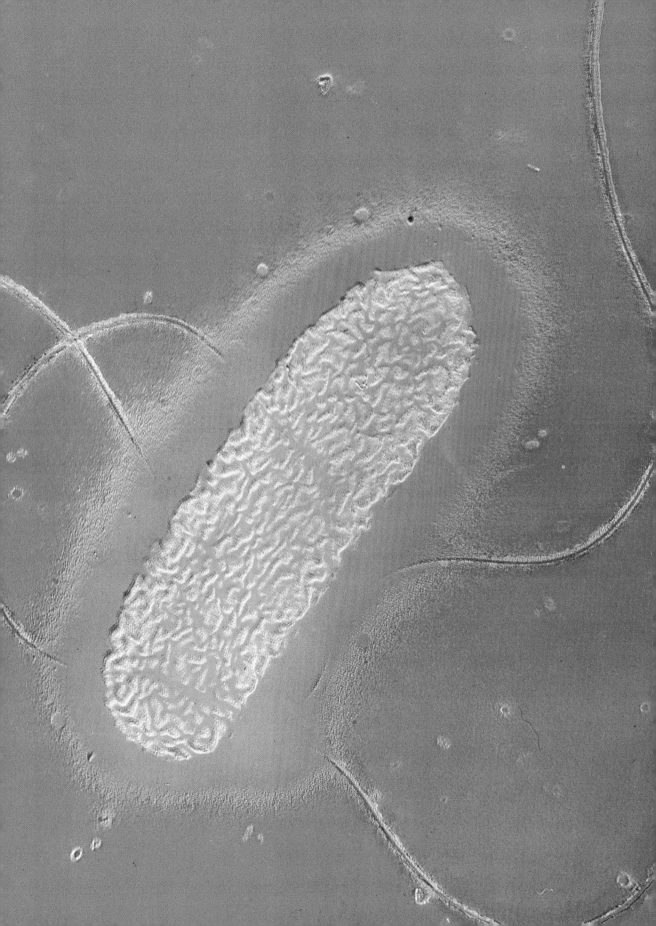

# PART TWO

# MATERIA MEDICA

Aconitum napellus (*Aconite*)
Aesculus hippocastanum
Allium cepa
Antimonium tartaricum (*Ant tart*)
Apis mellifica
Argentum nitricum
Arnica montana
Arsenicum album
Belladonna
Bryonia alba
Calcarea carbonica (*Calc carb*)
Calcarea phosphorica (*Calc phos*)
Calendula
Cantharis
Carbo vegetabilis (*Carbo veg*)
Causticum
Chamomilla
China officinalis
Cocculus indicus
Coccus cacti
Colocynthis
Dioscorea
Drosera
Eupatorium perfoliatum
Euphrasia
Ferrum phosphoricum (*Ferrum phos*)
Gelsemium
Hamamelis
Hepar sulphuris calcareum
    (*Hepar sulph*)

Hypericum
Ignatia
Ipecacuanha
Lachesis
Ledum palustre
Lycopodium
Magnesia phosphorica (*Mag phos*)
Mercurius
Natrum muriaticum (*Nat mur*)
Natrum sulphuricum (*Nat sulph*)
Nux Vomica
Phosphorus
Phytolacca
Podophyllum
Pulsatilla
Rhus toxicodendron (*Rhus tox*)
Rumex crispus
Ruta graveolens
Sabadilla
Sarsaparilla
Silica
Spongia
Staphysagria
Sulphur
Symphytum
Tabacum
Tarentula cubensis (*Tarent cub*)
Urtica urens
Veratrum album (*Veratrum alb*)
Verbascum
Rescue remedy

*Salmonella enteritidis (facing page) is a bacterium often associated with bad stomach upsets where symptoms include diarrhoea and vomiting. Arsenicum is usually the first remedy to try in such situations.*

## *Aconitum napellus*

Aconite is prepared from monkshood, a striking plant that grows in mountainous regions of Europe and Asia. It has a beautiful cluster of violet-blue flowers arranged like a monk's cowl. Its beauty belies its nature, however, for it is one of the most poisonous of plants. Homeopathy has a unique way of turning even this most toxic of substances into harmless but powerful medicines.

Almost everything about this remedy is sudden and violent. Symptoms appear without warning, especially at night. Often the cause is unknown, but it can be cold winds, draughts, or fright. Aconite is a remedy much associated with terror, fear, or at the least, extreme anxiety. Sufferers tend to be restless and emotionally wrought. Pains can take the form of intense burning or tingling. There can be a hot, bursting headache, like a band around the head. A high temperature is common, with burning thirst and a drenching sweat. It is a good remedy when a cough is hoarse, croupy, dry, and painful. Aconite states are made worse by light, noise, severe emotional turmoil, and cold. The sufferer needs rest and quiet. Fear is very marked and if the condition is severe the sufferer is sure he or she is going to die.

Aconite is a remedy that should be used at the beginning of an illness so prescribe it quickly. If you wait too long, the opportunity is lost and another remedy will be indicated.

## *Aesculus hippocastanum*

Aesculus is more popularly known as the horse chestnut tree. The remedy has a marked affinity with the veins of the lower bowel and rectum, which makes it a great haemorrhoid remedy. Aesculus produces a sensation of dry heat, stiffness, and roughness, when "proved" in the healthy person. Use it for piles that are noticeably purple and painful, with sharp pains shooting up the back. Sufferers feel worse for walking or standing. The remedy can either be taken internally or used as a cream.

## *Allium cepa*

Everyone knows the symptoms of this remedy, for we have all experienced the streaming eyes and nose caused by the red onion. It affects the mucous membranes of the nose, eyes, and larynx, causing violent sneezing and an acrid discharge from the nose. Although the eyes burn, the tears are bland. Its main uses are for head colds, tickling coughs, and hayfever. Symptoms ease in the cool open air.

## Antimonium tartaricum

Ant tart is prepared from tartar emetic, a chemical compound including antimony and potash. As its name suggests it used to be employed as an emetic. It greatly affects the mucous membranes of the lungs, where quantities of mucus accumulate. The remedy helps a weak person to cough up this phlegm and it helps the all-important spots in chickenpox or measles form properly. It is also an important remedy for nausea that may be accompanied by diarrhoea.

## Apis mellifica

Better known as the honey bee, Apis is a very important remedy for acute ailments. Its symptoms resemble the characteristics of the insect in its natural environment. Anyone who has watched a bee restlessly flitting from flower to flower gathering nectar, or who has experienced the swelling pain of the bee's sting, will have some knowledge of the symptoms of Apis. Further observations of the bee in its hive reveals groups of worker bees furiously fanning their wings to keep the hive cool in the hottest of summers. The queen bee meanwhile brooks no rivals and stings all other budding queens to death.

Mentally the keynotes are extreme restlessness and busyness, irritability, jealousy, and angry reactions to outside interference. There is extreme sensitivity to heat – all ailments are better for cool air or cold compresses. Pains are burning and stinging, and visible symptoms look shiny, red, puffy, and swollen – just like a bee sting. All symptoms develop rapidly, especially fevers, which tend to be thirstless despite the burning heat. The sufferer feels drowsy, but finds it difficult to sleep.

Most ailments showing the above symptoms will respond to Apis. Notable conditions include insect stings, fevers, cystitis, measles, mumps, and tonsillitis and swollen eyelids, lips, and tongue.

## Argentum nitricum

Arg nit is prepared from the crystalline salt, silver nitrate. This substance has long been known to medieval alchemists, but has a more modern use in the preparation of photographic film. Arg nit subjects are impressionable and rather nervous, with a tendency to hurry and worry. It is a great remedy for anticipation; for those people who dread ordeals.

The very thought of the exam, the plane flight, and so on, can cause them virtual paralysis with fear, which leads to diarrhoea and flatulence.

*Calcarea carbonica comes from lime in oyster shells (overleaf, left). Rhus tox (overleaf, right), better known as Poison Ivy, causes a severe rash if touched. The remedy derived from this plant is a major first-aid remedy for sprains.*

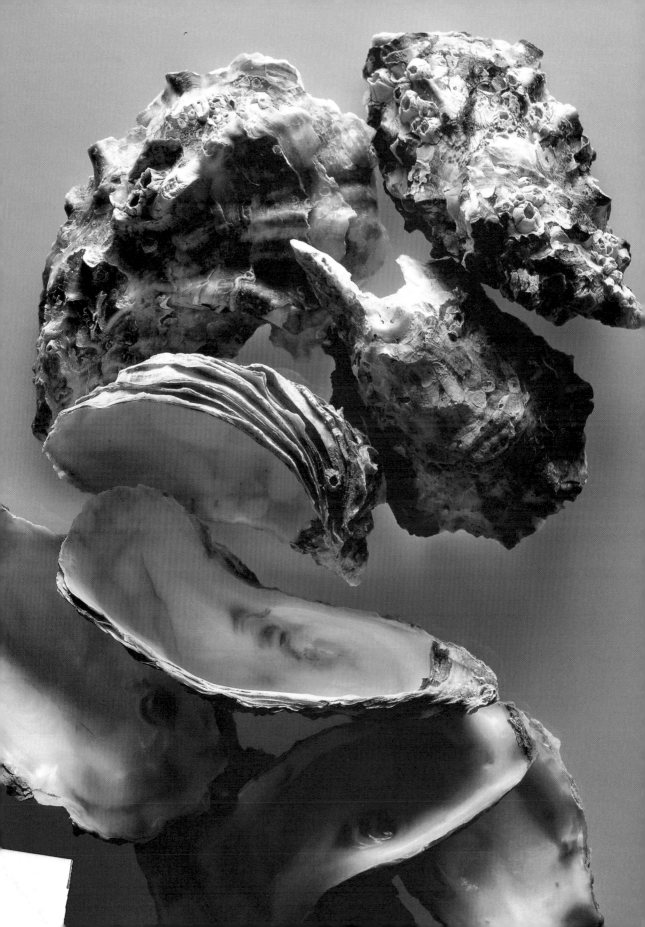

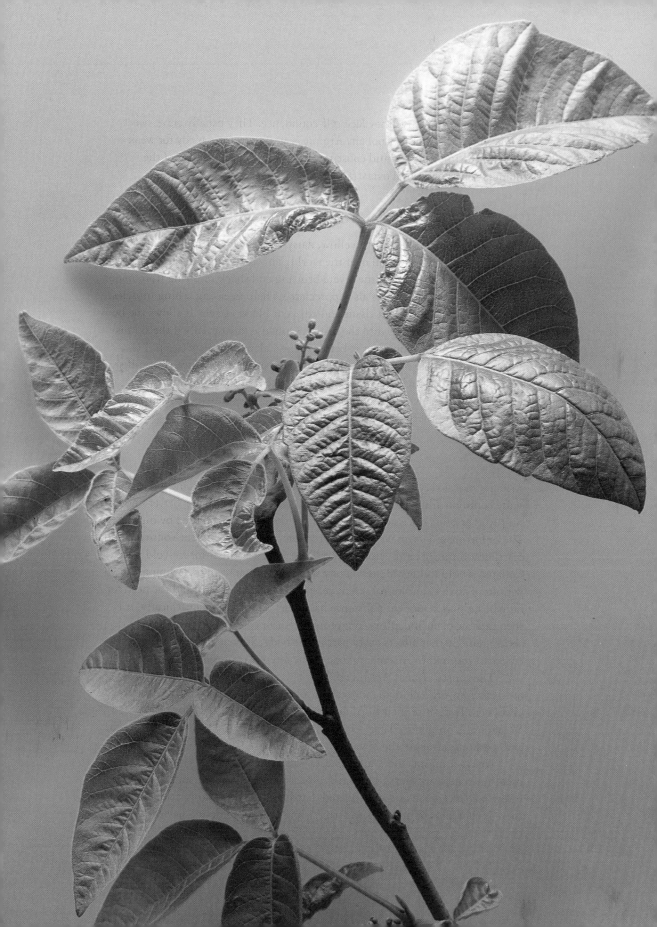

Though often impulsive they lack self-confidence. They usually crave sweet things and feel better for cool air. Arg nit is an important remedy for weak nerves resulting from a timid constitution, of some irrational fear of the moment, or from mental overstrain.

## Arnica montana

Arnica is a perennial herb with yellow, daisy-like flowers. It grows in cool, damp, mountainous areas all over the world. This is appropriate as Arnica is the most important remedy for the severe bruising and shock resulting from major falls and accidents. Climbers also appreciate its help in easing aching muscles.

Arnica acts on the soft tissue and adjacent blood vessels. It allows the body to reabsorb the blood lost into the bruise. Only use it externally if the skin is unbroken. For open wounds it is better to use Calendula cream (see p. 71). Shock is the keynote of the mental symptoms that call for Arnica. The sufferer cannot bear to be touch or even approached. Use Arnica for any injury or accident where bruising or shock is present. For minor bruises or strains apply it as a cream, but otherwise take it in pill form in the normal way.

## Arsenicum album

Arsenicum is a very important remedy for both long-term chronic diseases and acute common ailments. The natural substance arsenious oxide, better known simply as arsenic, has a notorious history as the main poison used by murderers. The unfortunate victim would die in terrible agony with violent vomiting and diarrhoea, burning pains, stomach cramps, and great thirst for ice-cold water. Collapse would follow. Mental agony was also pronounced, including great periods of anxiety and terror, an understandable fear of death, and the need for human support. Once the substance has been "tamed" homeopathically, it is then capable of curing all the symptoms mentioned above. Arsenicum is a deep-acting remedy that affects every part of the body. Stomach upsets, and gastro-enteritis, respond to Arsenicum; one of the foremost cures for this disease.

The constitutional Arsenicum type is very fastidious and tidy, rather oversensitive, critical, demanding, and restless. Arsenicum types are nearly always chilly despite their burning pains, which can be helped by heat. Weakness is pronounced and seems out of proportion to the disease. Midnight and the hours after are the lowest times.

Arsenicum can cure many diseases where the indicated symptoms mentioned here are marked, but it is especially useful for ailments of the gastro-intestinal tract, such as vomiting and diarrhoea; the respiratory tract, where there is shortness of breath as in asthma, and in head colds and hayfever.

## Belladonna

European parents have warned generations of children never to eat the large, poisonous berries of the tall plant appropriately named deadly nightshade, though Italian ladies of fashion found a way of putting this plant to cosmetic use during the Renaissance period; it enlarged their pupils. The plant became known as "belladonna", or beautiful lady.

Belladonna symptoms are intense and appear suddenly. They include fever with a high temperature, a burning, dry skin and mouth, yet surprisingly little thirst, although sometimes there is a craving for lemonade. There is also restlessness, and in extreme cases, delerium. The head or part of it, such as the ears, throat, tongue, or gums are almost always red. Intense pain throbs, like blood pounding through the veins. Belladonna can be a major headache remedy if the pain throbs like lots of little hammers and the face is bright red.

Generally, Belladonna ailments are exacerbated by sun and light, touch, pressure, and draughts. As in Aconite, it is most successfully used in the early stages of a disease. Consider it for any ailment that appears suddenly and that features the keynotes of burning heat, dryness, bright redness, and severe throbbing pain, especially in the head area.

## Bryonia alba

Bryonia is one of those extremely important remedies with many uses and a distinctive picture. It should be in everybody's first-aid kit (see p. 92). The remedy is derived from white bryony, a common climbing plant that grows throughout Europe. Its habit is to grow slowly and unobtrusively, which is how Bryonia ailments develop. This is an important symptom – the remedy is unlikely to be Bryonia if speed and drama are involved. The other important symptom is dryness that has several manifestations throughout the body – the respiratory airways, the digestive tract, or the joints. There seems to be a problem in lubrication and not surprisingly there is a marked thirst for long draughts of cold water.

If the respiratory tract is affected there will be a dry, hard, very painful cough that may feel easier for holding the chest. In bronchitis or asthma there may be stitching pains in the chest. Dryness in the stomach and intestines leads to a sluggish digestion with very hard, large, dry stools. The lack of lubrication makes the sufferer want to keep very still; the slightest movement causes pain and hard pressure eases it. The sufferer's manner is "dry" as well; s/he is grumpy and irritable, wants to be left alone, and to go home if not already there. There are few ailments that Bryonia cannot help if the above symptoms indicate. The more common ones, however, include coughs, colds, bronchitis, influenza, stomach upsets, headaches, joint pains, mumps, and measles.

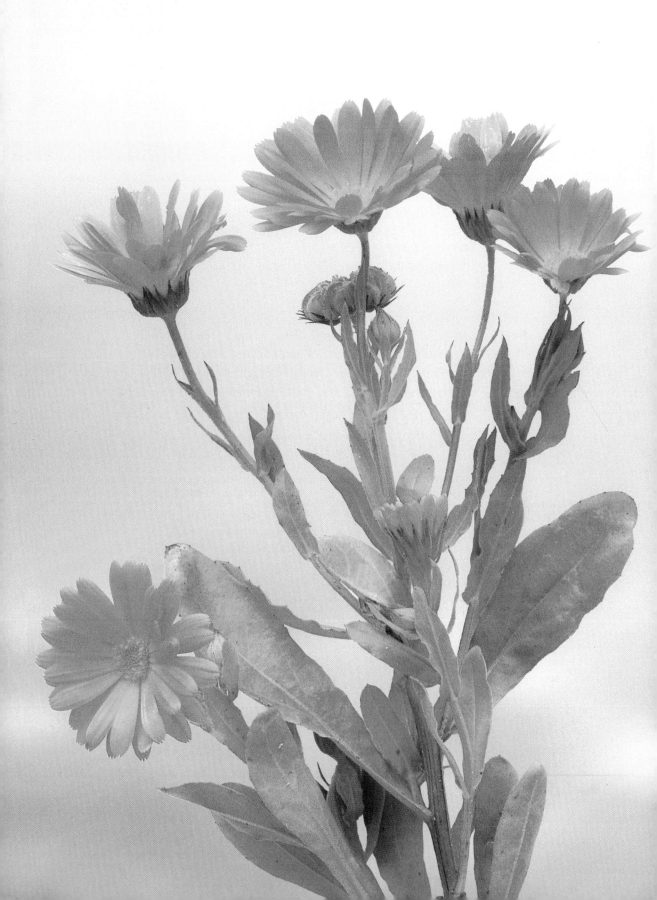

## Calcarea carbonica

Calc carb, as it is usually known, is primarily a constitutional and chronic remedy rather than a day-to-day acute one. It is one of the main childhood remedies described in some detail on page 53. Calc carb is lime, a compound of calcium and carbon; the homeopathic remedy is derived from the middle layer of the shell of the oyster, which is a particularly pure source. Calcium is one of the most important elements in the body, notably in the bones, and is an essential building block for growth and nutrition. It is a remedy with many uses, but its main indicators are in the mental sphere. These include slowness and stubbornness, and an oversensitivity that gives rise to a great many fears.

Physically the Calc carb subject tends to be on the plump side and rather out of condition; a sweaty head and sweaty hands are characteristic. The remedy's prescription is generally best left to the homeopathic practitioner, although parents can try it on their children, if symptoms indicate it, and if they fit the constitutional type description.

## Calcarea phosphorica

Calc phos is a mineral containing calcium and phosphorus, the main constituent elements of bone. It has an important role in bone repair and nutrition. Use it for the aftermath of a fracture, once Symphytum has been used to knit the bones (see p. 89), and for people whose bones are soft, thin, and brittle. Calc phos also helps the growing pains of children, especially those who are tall and thin, and are prone to headaches and swollen glands.

## Calendula

Calendula is a herb known to almost everybody; it is a species of marigold, a small, annual flowering plant with deep-orange flowers. It is the most important remedy for healing open wounds, ranging from simple cuts to major injuries. Calendula not only speeds up healing but also prevents wounds from becoming septic. For small injuries it is easier to use as a cream, although diluted tincture (one part to ten parts of water) will serve just as well. For more serious injuries take it in pill form in addition.

*Calendula (facing page) provides a major first-aid remedy for cuts and sores.*

## Cantharis

Cantharis is prepared from a small, brilliant-green beetle, known as Spanish fly. It is excellent for burning pains, where the sufferer feels "on fire". Cantharis is therefore an important first-aid remedy for minor burns and scalds, where blistering and inflammation occur (see p. 28), as well as for sunburn and insect bites, where burning is the predominant symptom. It has an affinity with the urinary tract, making it a very important remedy in the treatment of cystitis. Cantharis symptoms develop suddenly. There may also be a burning thirst.

## Carbo vegetabilis

Carbo veg is a charcoal preparation that has an affinity with the circulation and its oxygen content. It is an important remedy in collapse, where the sufferer desperately needs oxygen and fresh air, but does not have the strength to obtain it. Coldness, weakness, paleness, and flatulence are important symptoms. It is used more as a chronic remedy and is best prescribed by a homeopathic practitioner.

## Causticum

Causticum is a curious mixture of slaked lime and potassium bisulphate invented by Hahnemann himself (see p. 8). It is an important chronic and constitutional remedy with a marked affinity to the nervous system and mind, as well as the neuro-muscular system. It is also useful for coughs and hoarseness resulting from over use of the voice. Like Cantharis (see above) it is a major burn remedy in first aid.

## Chamomilla

Chamomilla is a member of the daisy family and grows wild all over Europe. It strongly affects the nervous system, causing extreme irritability and oversensitivity to pain. These symptoms must be present to indicate Chamomilla.

Its most famous use is for bad-tempered teething babies for whom nothing pleases and who throw their toys across the room in an angry manner. Relief only comes from being carried or rocked. (It is not, though, exclusively a children's remedy.) Use it for colic; the baby's stools may smell like rotten eggs and look like slimy, chopped-up spinach. Pain is often worse at night and the temper is exacerbated by being looked at, spoken to, or touched. In children, one cheek may look pale while the other is red, but sometimes they are both red.

## China officinalis

China is prepared from the bark of the Quinaquina, a tree that grows high in the Andes mountains. It was the first remedy actually "proved" by the founder of homeopathy, Hahnemann (see p. 8). It affects the blood and circulation and is a remedy for extreme weakness from loss of vital fluids such as in haemorrhage or diarrhoea. It is also an important remedy for fevers with drenching sweat, as in malaria. China is a chronic remedy with strong mental symptoms; it is best prescribed by a homeopathic practitioner in chronic cases.

## Cocculus indicus

Cocculus, or the Indian cockle, is a plant that grows along the coasts of India. It strongly affects the central nervous system and is a remedy for exhaustion when the sufferer feels worn out. Although it has several other uses, the remedy can help with the nausea and vomiting that arises from travel sickness, as the sufferer is affected by the motion of boats, trains, cars, or even swimming.

## Coccus cacti

Coccus cacti, or cochineal, is a remedy prepared from a Central American insect that feeds off the prickly pear. It has a specific action on the mucous membranes of the throat. There is extreme irritation causing paroxysms of violent, tickling coughing, raising clear, ropy mucus that hangs out of the mouth. The sufferer feels hot and has a red face. Coccus cacti is a splendid remedy for whooping cough with these symptoms.

## Colocynthis

Colocynthis, or bitter cucumber, is a gourd that grows in hot, dry regions of Asia and Africa. Extreme bad temper is an important characteristic of this remedy, whatever the ailment. As well as the nerves the remedy has an impact on the stomach and digestive tract. The pains in this area are violent and cutting, and are better for hard pressure and doubling up. The remedy is very helpful for stomach upsets and colic, where these symptoms are prominent.

## Dioscorea

Dioscorea, or wild yam, is a creeper that grows in hedges and woods in North America. It is a very important remedy for abdominal cramps or colic in babies. It acts on the nerves and helps with the sharp, agonizing, twisting pains. The pain improves by stretching out or bending backward.

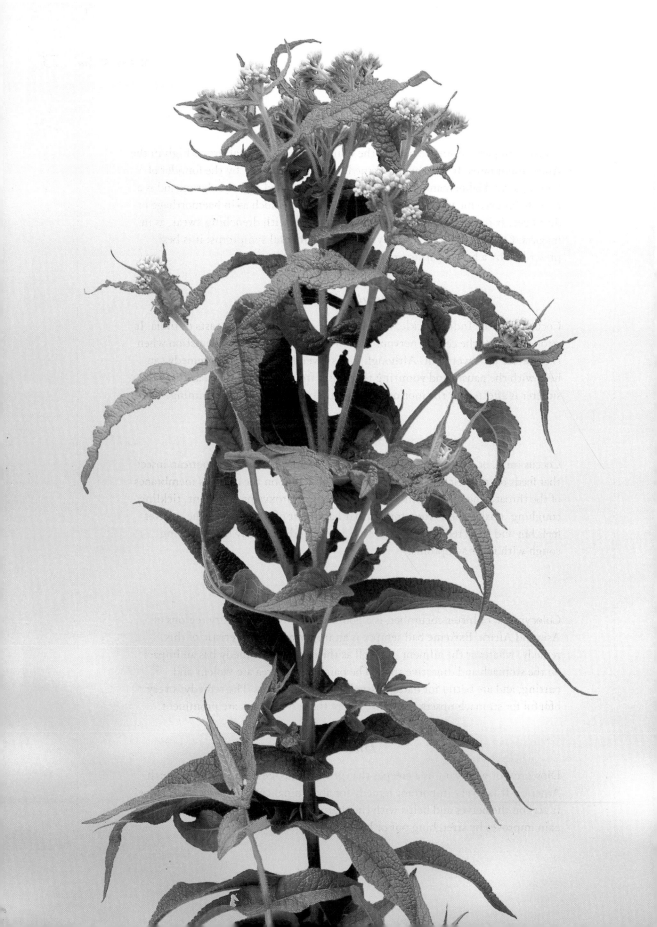

### Drosera

Drosera, or round-leafed sundew, is an extraordinary plant found growing in the marshes and bogs of the northern hemisphere. The plant secretes a sticky fluid that assists in trapping any careless insect that alights on it. The insect is then drawn within and devoured. Drosera affects the respiratory organs and is a major cough remedy. The deep, barking cough is a prolonged and incessant one, with choking coming on in periodic fits. It is usually worse after midnight and for lying down. Symptoms that accompany the cough include retching and vomiting, breathlessness, nosebleeds, and sweating. It is an important remedy in the treatment of whooping cough.

### Eupatorium perfoliatum

Eupatorium, or boneset, is a well-known herb that grows in damp places in North America. It is aptly named for it helps in colds and influenza where the pain seems to have penetrated deep into the bones. The pain is quite violent and has been described as "bone breaking". The muscles of the chest, back, and limbs often feel sore and bruised. There will also be nausea, possibly followed by vomiting of bile. The sufferer will be very thirsty and feverish, and there may be a painful cough.

### Euphrasia

Also known as eyebright, Euphrasia is a traditional remedy for sore and inflamed eyes. It is a small, delicate meadow plant with white, purple, and yellow multicoloured flowers that open wide in the sunshine. The eyes freely water with acrid secretions. If the nose is affected, its discharge is bland. Symptoms are worse for sunlight, wind, and warmth, and better for the open air. Use in cases of hayfever and colds, where the eyes are the main area affected.

### Ferrum phosphoricum

Ferrum phos is a mineral compound of iron and phosphorus and is mainly used for influenza and fevers. Symptoms tend not to be clear and obvious, but are best described as a slight temperature, general tiredness, and head cold. Use Ferrum phos for violent earache if Belladonna (see p. 69) is indicated but does not work. Symptoms usually develop slowly.

*Eupatorium (facing page). This North American plant produces a major 'flu remedy.*

### Gelsemium

Gelsemium, the yellow jasmine of North America, not to be confused with the yellow winter jasmine, is a source of one of the most important acute remedies for influenza in the Materia Medica. It acts primarily on the muscles and their motor nerves. The muscles ache, feel extremely heavy, and there is a feeling of chilliness and overwhelming weakness and tiredness. It feels as if the mind no longer seems to control the body; even the eyelids droop. Symptoms develop slowly and when there is fever the sufferer sweats, though drinks little. There may be also dizziness, a watery discharge from the nose, and a dull heavy headache that is often concentrated at the back of the head. There is an inclination to urinate profusely, with a feeling of relief afterwards. Shivering or trembling is almost always predominant, whatever the ailment.

Gelsemium is also of great assistance as an anticipation remedy. There is a great fear of ordeals, such as exams, public speaking, interviews, or meeting important people. As in influenza the keynote is trembling; the knees may actually knock together or the hands shake with fear while thinking about, or enduring, the event.

### Hamamelis

Hamamelis is more commonly known as witch hazel, a small North American tree. It has a marked action on the veins, especially in the limbs and in the areas of the rectum and throat. It is therefore an important remedy for varicose veins and haemorrhoids. Veins feel bruised, painful, and sore, and look swollen and inflamed. It is a good remedy for varicose veins arising from pregnancy. For haemorrhoids that bleed profusely, use it locally as a cream, or internally.

### Hepar sulphuris calcareum

Hepar sulph is a complex mixture of calcium and sulphur prepared from combining lime from oyster shells and sulphur. It has a strong affinity with the nerves and Hepar sulph types are famed for their bad temper and general oversensitivity to all external impressions. These include noise, cold and draughts, touch, and the slightest pain. The pain feels like a sharp splinter: the same sensation as a fishbone stuck in the throat. There is heavy sweating with a sour smell. Sufferers feel the cold so much that they insist on keeping extremely well "wrapped-up", especially the head, which they like to be covered. Strangely, dampness helps their condition – as long as it is warm.

The remedy is important for septic states, such as in abscesses where pus has built up to the point of discharging and may actually be oozing out. This

smells very offensive – like old cheese. Hepar sulph is also a major cough and croup remedy. The cough is hoarse and worse for cold. There is a lot of thick, yellow mucus that is difficult to shift from the chest. Sour foods and drink are sometimes craved.

Hepar sulph can ease or cure a whole battery of ailments. These include earache, toothache, coughs, bronchitis, and laryngitis. Use the remedy for injuries, abscesses, and boils that fester and will not heal. The main keynotes are irritability and anger, extreme chilliness, sweatiness, infection with pus present, and sharp pains. If all these are present, then Hepar sulph should help.

## Hypericum

Hypericum, or St John's wort, is a well-known and traditional herb growing throughout Europe and Asia. It is basically an injury remedy with an affinity to the parts of the body rich in sensitive nerves. These areas include the fingers and toes, lips, ears and eyes, and the coccyx region of the spine. The pains follow the tracts of the nerves and are often experienced as shooting pains. Hypericum can be used either as a cream or diluted tincture (one part to ten parts water), or internally for more severe injuries.

## Ignatia

Ignatia is a remedy prepared from St Ignatius' bean, a beautiful tree found in the Philippines and China. The remedy is obtained from the bitter seeds, which produce strange effects on the mind and emotions, including trembling, twitching, cramps, giddiness, nervousness, terrible dreams, sadness, and despair. Symptoms are contradictory and perverse – you never quite know where you stand with someone who needs Ignatia. The sufferer experiences changeable moods, laughing and crying by turns, is extremely emotional, given to deep brooding, seemingly lost in his or her own little world of grief and melancholy. It is, in fact, a very important remedy for grief and emotional loss, and the after-effects of grief. Ignatia eases the pain of many other emotional ailments, if they are unusually prolonged. These include fright, humiliation, worry, shock, and anger, especially when they are hidden and locked away inside. Look for pronounced sighing as an outward sign. Another symptom is a feeling of a lump in the throat that cannot be swallowed. These sufferers are also sensitive physically and may be made worse by coffee, tobacco smoke, or being touched. During headaches, it feels as if a nail is actually being hammered in. The stomach can feel empty even after eating. Ignatia can cure numerous ailments that seem to have an emotional underlay.

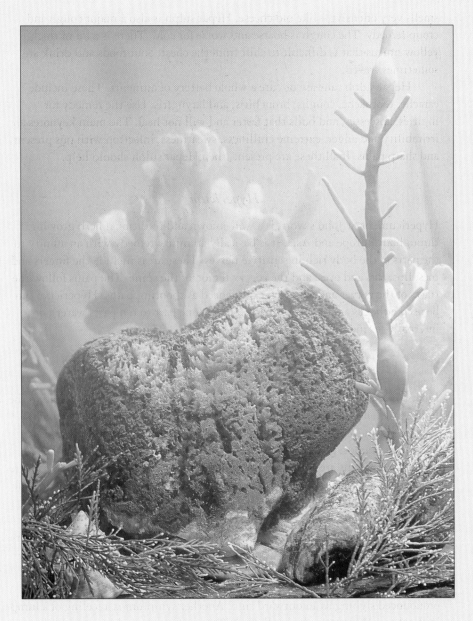

***Spongia****. The marine sponge when roasted and dried is the source of a major cough remedy. It is also an important remedy for croup in children.*

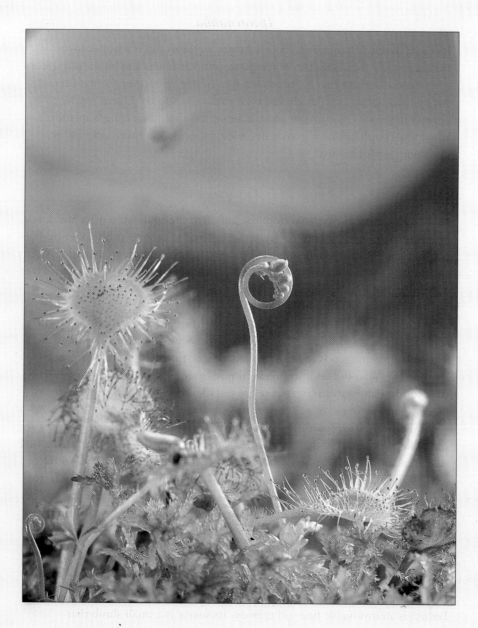

***Drosera***. *The Round-leafed Sundew, an extraordinary insect-eating plant, gives us a useful cough remedy. The cough comes in paroxysms that take the breath away.*

## *Ipecacuanha*

Ipecac is derived from a small South American shrub and is a well-known nausea remedy. It acts on the whole gastro-intestinal area and on the respiratory tract. Ipecac is also a notable haemorrhage remedy. Whatever the symptoms, strong nausea, not usually relieved by vomiting, has to be present for the remedy to work. The ailments include headache, diarrhoea, coughs including whooping cough, asthma, gastric flu, fever, influenza, morning sickness in pregnancy – plus nausea.

## *Lachesis*

Lachesis is a remedy prepared from the poison of the South American Surukuku, or bushmaster snake. About seven feet long (2m), the snake kills its victims by poisoning and constriction and, unlike most snakes, is considered to be very aggressive. The poison is homeopathically diluted and succussed into one of the most powerful healing medicines. Lachesis is a remedy no homeopathic practitioner can afford to be without.

It is a remedy used for chronic and constitutional cases rather than for common ailments, but it can be very helpful in acute infections of the throat. The inflammation tends to be on the left side, or moves from left to right. Swallowing is painful and, strangely, liquids may be more difficult to swallow than solids. Pains can stretch to the ear and the throat and neck area can be so tender that wearing a collar or any restriction feels like torture.

Many of the symptoms and characteristics of the chronic Lachesis type resemble, if not exactly the snake, at least the wilder, passionate, and instinctual side of mankind. Lachesis personalities do not like restraints – they are often jealous, loquacious, suspicious, and oversensitive individuals. They are affected badly by heat and any pressure, especially around the neck, chest, or waist. They are at their worst upon waking. It is an important female remedy and as it has an affinity with the ovaries is particularly useful around the time of the menopause.

## *Ledum palustre*

Ledum is an invaluable first-aid remedy. Its source is a small shrub that looks rather like the tea plant; it is sometimes known as marsh tea. The plant grows in cold, damp bogs and marshes in northern Europe and northern America. Its main use is for puncture wounds from sharp points or insect stings and bites. The resulting injury does not heal well; feels strangely cold to the touch and looks purple and puffy. You can help the pain by cold compresses. Ledum is also a remedy for bloodshot eyes.

## *Lycopodium*

Lycopodium is one of the major polycrests: a remedy with numerous uses. The plant, club moss, grows on heaths in Europe and North America. It is extraordinary to look at; a long, straggling, prostrate plant many yards long, regularly pushing up stems like aerials. The dried spores from which the remedy is prepared do not absorb water and were once used in fireworks.

Largely prescribed as a deep constitutional or chronic remedy for all ages it acts very deeply on the digestive system (see page 54 for a detailed description of the symptoms). Lycopodium types very often have weak digestions with heartburn and flatulence and abnormal distortions in the appetite, aggravated by gassy foods such as beans and cabbages. There is usually a craving for sweets. There is also an affinity with the urinary system and its ailments. Lycopodium subjects classically wake up cross in the morning and have a low point between 4pm and 8pm. The pressure of tight clothes and a stuffy atmosphere causes intense discomfort. Mentally Lycopodiums lack self-confidence and are big worriers, but can cover it up by being domineering and dictatorial. Lycopodiums enjoy undemanding relationships as they tend to live in their heads, but like someone around for security.

Lycopodium is not used so much in common ailments, but as it is mainly a right-sided remedy consider it for sore throats that start on, or stay on, the right side. Use it as a remedy for anticipatory fears, if other symptoms support it.

## *Magnesia phosphorica*

Mag phos, a simple compound of magnesium and phosphorus, has a direct effect on the nerves and muscles. It is a wonderful remedy for neuralgic pains and cramps. Pains tend to appear in violent paroxysms and shoot like lightning. Being worse at night and exacerbated by cold and draughts, warmth and pressure relieves them. The use of a hot-water bottle or doubling up in the case of stomach cramps eases the pains. Mag phos is a remedy for colic, menstrual cramps, sciatica, toothache, and earache.

## *Mercurius*

Mercurius, or Mercury, as it is commonly known, was formerly used in very large doses as a medicine for syphilis. Such were the side effects that the disease was probably preferable to the cure. Mercury has a more modern use in the thermometer and Mercury types seem to have problems with their inner thermostat, suffering from extremes of heat and cold. Mercury has a well-defined symptom picture and is used for both chronic diseases and in more acute conditions of common ailments. It strongly affects the glands and their

secretions. The glands are swollen and their over-activity produces increased saliva, worse at night, and a wet, flabby, yellowish tongue that shows the imprint of the teeth. Sweat is a major symptom, accompanied by thirst. The breath is offensive and there can be a metallic taste in the mouth.

Mercury is a remedy for septic states, so it is very useful for boils and abscesses. Discharges are often blood-streaked and are more profuse and more painful at night. Patients tend to be exhausted, irritable, and restless, and children who need it constitutionally may be mischievous and dictatorial.

Mercury is useful for many ailments, including sore throats and tonsillitis, earache, mouth ulcers and toothache, chickenpox, and mumps. Any ailment that has predominant symptoms of sweating and thirst, increased saliva, and offensiveness of secretions and discharges can benefit from Mercurius.

## *Natrum muriaticum*

Nat mur is sodium chloride, or common salt and it is one of the most important remedies. Salt is essential to life, regulating the fluids and flow of vital minerals throughout the body. Similarly the remedy Nat mur affects the water balance and has an affinity with the nutrition and mucous membranes, as well as deeply affecting the emotions and the mind. Its main use is in chronic conditions and it is not so often used in acute ones (see page 56 for a description of Nat mur as a child's constitutional remedy). Many of its most important symptoms are connected with the feelings, and notably with ones that are not easily expressed. These include grief, rejection, buried resentment, and humiliation. Usually Nat mur subjects have difficulty crying, but sometimes the reverse is true – being unable to stop weeping. They prefer to be alone and dislike being consoled in a crisis. Oversensitive to criticism they try to avoid any emotional pain, keeping their feelings to themselves. They dislike the hot sun, which may give them headaches, and experience a low time around 10am. They often crave salt and can be very thirsty. Nat mur types are also prone to headaches, palpitations, and cold sores.

## *Natrum sulphuricum*

Nat sulph, or sodium sulphate, is also known as Glauber's salt and was used in material doses for constipation. As a homeopathic remedy it does the opposite, helping to cure extremely loose stools and flatulence. It is important for ailments caused by damp – such as asthma. Nat sulph is an important remedy for the liver and is sometimes used for problems following head injuries.

*Hypericum (facing page), or St John's Wort, as this herb is commonly known, is an important first-aid remedy for injuries.*

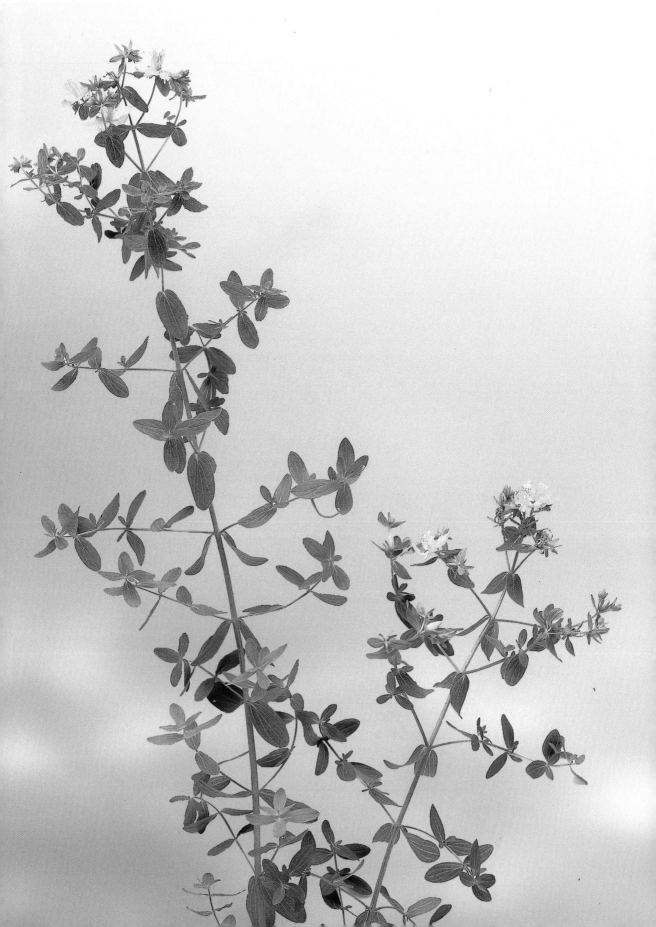

### *Nux vomica*

Nux vomica is obtained from the poison nut tree, a native of the Far East. It is a major medicine for both chronic and acute situations, most notably in disturbances of the digestion such as violent vomiting and nausea or when there is a great desire to vomit without being able to. Similarly, there is a great need to pass a stool, but the urging can be fruitless, or the result unsatisfactory. There may be alternate diarrhoea and constipation. Food lies like a heavy load in the stomach and is slow to digest. It is a good heartburn remedy when there are watery and sour risings.

Overindulgence is often the cause – Nux vomica types are prone to eating too much rich food and consuming a lot of alcohol. The remedy has gained some recognition as a hangover remedy and it also suits the workaholic who has too many business lunches, who is irritable, oversensitive, and impatient, and is always worrying about work. Nux vomica types tend to be tidy and fastidious people, and there is great sensitivity underneath the touchiness. They would feel much better if they could "loosen up", both mentally and physically – their tight clothing hurts the stomach – eat and drink less, and take more exercise. It is very much a 20th-century medicine.

Nux vomica is a remedy for chilly people who catch cold easily; who wake too early and cannot get back to sleep again. It can be used for all sorts of ailments including ulcers, coughs, influenza, headaches, sore throats, and earache, provided that the general symptom picture above fits.

### *Phosphorus*

The element phosphorus is an essential constituent of animal and vegetable life and was first isolated from urine. It is found throughout the body, but there is a concentration in the bones and the homeopathic preparation is derived from the phosphorus found in bone ash. The element is very volatile when exposed to air and has to be stored under water for safety reasons. Homeopathically, Phosphorus types likewise tend to be extrovert and excitable, reacting enthusiastically to external events and impressions, although in sickness they are often quite the opposite, becoming dull and apathetic.

The typical Phosphorus child is described in the section dealing with children (see p. 57), but the description can equally apply to adults. Phosphorus is a particularly important remedy used in both chronic and acute prescribing. It can cure all manner of chronic ills if the constitutional Phosphorus temperament fits. Phosphorus people tend to be on the lively and open side, albeit somewhat nervous and anxious, and needing reassurance from others. Phosphorus has an affinity with the stomach and intestines and is an excellent remedy for ailments of the gastro-intestinal tract, such as vomiting, diarrhoea,

and general stomach problems. It is also a major respiratory remedy, especially suitable for people with "weak" chests who are prone to coughs and bronchitis. Phosphorus helps to clot the blood and is therefore useful in minor haemorrhages such as persistent nose bleeds.

## *Phytolacca*

Phytolacca, known as pokeroot in North America, is a small shrub found growing in damp places throughout the northern hemisphere. It affects the glands, especially the mammary glands and the tonsils, which feel, or appear, hard and sore. Phytolacca is therefore very useful for sore throats and in tonsillitis. Another major use is for mastitis and sore or cracked nipples.

## *Podophyllum*

Podophyllum is prepared from a North American herb also known as May apple, or mandrake. It is a small remedy and chiefly affects the duodenum and intestines, especially the rectum. Its main use is for chronic diarrhoea that is extraordinarily profuse and watery, and gushes out painlessly.

## *Pulsatilla*

Pulsatilla is another of those all-important remedies that neither the professional nor the lay prescriber can afford to be without. Its source is a beautiful purple bell-like flower of the anemone family known as the pasque flower, or windflower. It grows on chalk lands throughout north and central Europe. The flower tends to grow in groups, reminding us of one of the main themes of the constitutional Pulsatilla type – dependency. It is described in more detail under the children's section (see p. 60), but most of what is described there equally applies to adults. Pulsatilla is an important emotional remedy, sometimes called the weather-cock remedy, as people who need it suffer from ever-changing feelings and moods. It is often prescribed on the personality alone. Pulsatilla types are markedly yielding and gentle, and tend to be sensitive and weepy. They usually drink little, are warm-blooded, and feel very much better for being in fresh air. There are many ailments that will respond if the Pulsatilla picture fits. Its gentle, sympathetic nature, however, usually means that women will need it more often than men. Pulsatilla has so many uses that it would be impossible to list them all, but not surprisingly, it would include many female complaints such as period pains, varicose veins, and cystitis; all the children's basic ailments; colds and influenza (Pulsatilla discharges are yellow-green); gastro-intestinal ills (Pulsatillas should avoid rich, fatty foods), or any ailment where the symptoms constantly change.

### *Rhus toxicodendron*

The source of Rhus tox is a rambling North American plant, also known as poison ivy. Just to touch the leaves can bring up a very red and extremely itchy rash, which can lead to fever, joint pains, and swollen glands. Above all there is an intense restlessness. Like curing like, these are some of the symptoms to look for in sufferers needing Rhus tox. One keynote is initial stiffness in the joints that eases after gentle exercise. The remedy, therefore, can be very helpful in rheumatism, although it should not be used without taking all the sufferer's symptoms into account, because rheumatism can be a deep-seated disease.

Rhus tox is a very important first-aid remedy for sprains and strains, where the pain and stiffness improve from gentle motion. Complaints are better for warmth and massage, and worse for cold and damp, and over-exertion. It can be an excellent remedy in ailments such as chickenpox and shingles, where the rash is markedly itchy and the sufferer is extremely restless with it. Mentally the patient, not surprisingly, can be very sad and despondent. Sometimes a triangular red tip can be seen on the tongue. Often there is a thirst for large quantities of cold water or milk. Rhus tox is a major remedy that can cure very many ailments if the symptoms outlined above are marked.

### *Rumex crispus*

Rumex, or yellow dock, is a wayside weed found growing in Europe and North America. It has a marked affinity with the nerves, but more noticeably with the mucous membranes of the larynx and throat pit. Rumex, therefore, is an important cough remedy. The cough is worse for inhaling cold air and better for warmth and for covering the mouth. The cold air causes tickling in the throat, as if a feather were present. The constant irritation causes a dry, teasing cough, often worse at night.

### *Ruta graveolens*

Ruta is prepared from rue, a plant grown in herbal gardens since antiquity and well known for its action on tired eyes and for its first-aid qualities. Ruta has an affinity with the joints, tendons, cartilages, and the periosteum (the membrane that surrounds the bones). It is, therefore, an excellent remedy for bruised bones and injuries to the tendons, especially in the ankles and wrists. There is some restlessness, but not as much as in Rhus tox (see above), the other great remedy for sprains and strains.

*Ruta (facing page) was grown by monks in their monastic gardens. One of its uses was to relieve their eyes from the strain of writing illuminated manuscripts.*

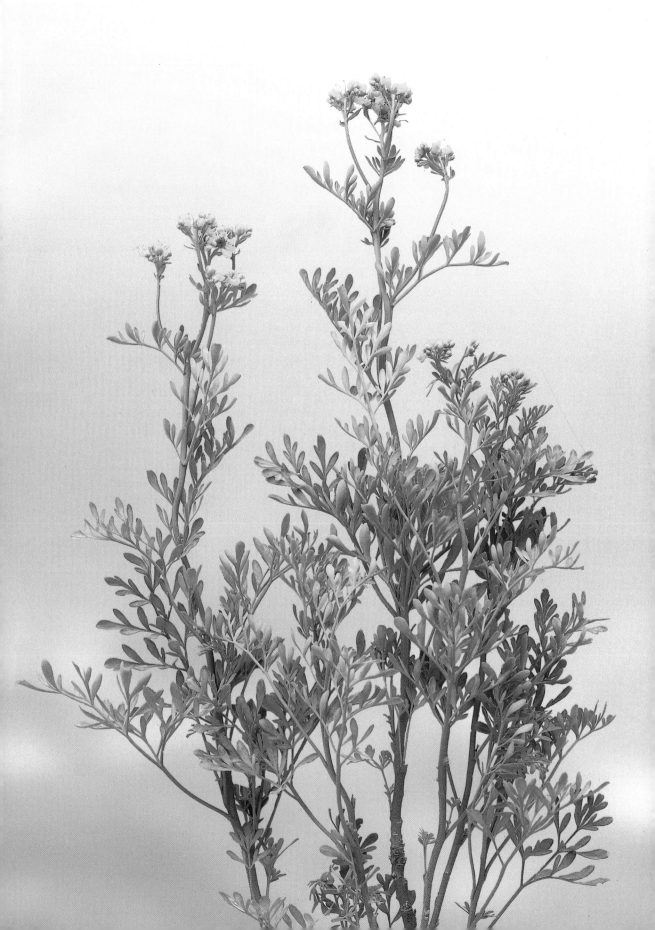

## Sabadilla

Sabadilla is prepared from the seeds of the cebadilla plant found growing in Mexico. The remedy particularly affects the mucous membranes of the nose. There is violent sneezing and itching; the nose feels stuffy and dry, though with a fluent discharge, and is oversensitive to pollen or dust. It is used to ease the discomfort of hayfever.

## Sarsaparilla

Sarsaparilla, or smilax, grows in North America. The remedy acts primarily on the genito-urinary organs and is mainly used as a cystitis remedy. Urination is very painful, although there is a constant urge, and can only be passed slowly. The distinguishing feature of Sarsaparilla is that the pain is particularly bad at the close of urination – the sufferer may even scream with agony.

## Silica

Homeopathic Silica is prepared from flint or sand. Silicon is one of the most abundant elements and essential to the supportive structure of plants. Silica is a major constitutional remedy that is used more often in chronic prescribing than for acute common ailments. As it is capable of expelling or reabsorbing diseased tissue it is excellent in the treatment of abscesses and boils that linger without coming to a head. Silica will also help push out foreign bodies, such as splinters, pieces of glass, or grit. Chronic Silica patients tend to be rather nervous, fearing sudden noises and bangs; the cold affects them badly and they lack self-confidence. They feel weak and tired, and have not the stamina to cope with life, finding it difficult to stick up for themselves. Children who need it may have defective nutrition, are slow growers, and find it hard to put on weight. Poor concentration and an obstinate personality affects their progress at school.

## Spongia

The roasted and powdered skeleton of the Mediterranean sponge produces an effective homeopathic remedy. Spongia has an affinity with the heart and respiratory tract. It is used to treat coughs and croup. The cough is dry and hollow coming in fits, and sounds like a saw going through board. Cold and exertion make it worse.

## *Staphysagria*

Staphysagria, also known as larkspur or stavesacre, is a member of the delphinium family. It is a remedy for people who have suppressed their feelings of anger, grief, or indignation. They suffer in silence but, may be bubbling over inside. For this reason it is sometimes called the "civil servant's remedy". Such people are oversensitive and easily offended. They have difficulty saying no, and then feel used.

On a physical level Staphysagria is an excellent remedy for very sensitive cuts and wounds, especially when the patient has a feeling of having been humiliated or even violated, such as after an episiotomy or insensitive surgery.

## *Sulphur*

A natural chemical, Sulphur has been used for over 3000 years. It looks like yellow chalk and burns with suffocating fumes and has been associated with burning and purifying. It is present in spa water and in volcanic depths. Also called brimstone, it was once considered a main constituent of hell fire. Sulphur is basically a constitutional and chronic remedy and not used very much in the treatment of acute ailments. There have been more symptoms produced in its "provings" than any other remedy and it has a huge range of curative applications. Affecting every part of the body, it is an extremely deep-acting remedy, improving the circulation and metabolism, and the removal of toxins. Echoing a volcanic eruption, it brings things to the surface. For this reason it has long been associated with skin diseases. A description of the typical Sulphur child is included in the children's section (see p. 61) and much of this can be applied to the adult. One description of the archetypal Sulphur personality is "the ragged philosopher", living in his head without noticing his surroundings or even his own clothes. On a more physical level the Sulphur type has a low time around 11am, when a snack is needed to keep the energy up. He or she often has a sweet tooth and is usually warm-blooded, not noticing the cold.

## *Symphytum*

Symphytum, or comfrey, is a herb found growing in Europe, Asia, and North America. Its other name, knitbone, sums up its main use, which is to help heal broken bones. Once the fracture has been set, Symphytum speeds up the knitting of the bones together. It is also valuable for treating eye injuries.

## Tabacum

The nicotine in tobacco causes a deathly pale face and overwhelming nausea, sometimes followed by vomiting. The homeopathic equivalent, Tabacum, cures these symptoms. Tabacum is one of the main remedies for all kinds of motion sickness. The sufferer sweats profusely and feels better for cool, fresh air.

## Tarentula cubensis

The poison taken from a spider found in Cuba is the basis of Tarent cub. Use the remedy for boils or similar septic conditions that resemble the effects of the bite of this spider. Initial incubation is slow, but then it develops rapidly and alarmingly. There is terrible burning and the affected part is hard and purple.

## Urtica urens

Urtica, or the small stinging nettle, is a herb found growing throughout the world. It is a small remedy used mainly for minor burns and insect bites. It is useful in the treatment of hives and prickly heat. Urtica affects the mammary glands and helps increase the supply of milk in breastfeeding mothers.

## Veratrum album

White hellebore, the herb from which Veratrum alb is prepared, grows in the mountains of central Europe. It has a well-defined chronic picture and is also a well-known remedy for violent diarrhoea and vomiting. Veratrum alb is a major cholera remedy. Apart from the continuous vomiting and diarrhoea the sufferer feels extremely cold and weak, with an unquenchable thirst for ice-cold water.

## Verbascum

Verbascum is normally used as an oil prepared from the common mullein, a plant found all over Europe and North America. Having a very soothing effect in the ears, Verbascum oil is an excellent remedy to use in earache. Use only a few warmed drops.

## Rescue remedy

The Bach Flower Rescue or First-Aid Remedy is not really a homeopathic medicine, but a combination of five of the well-known flower remedies. It should be used in conjunction with any normal homeopathic remedy in times of crisis or shock.

*Symphytum (facing page), otherwise known as Comfrey, helps to knit fractured bones together.*

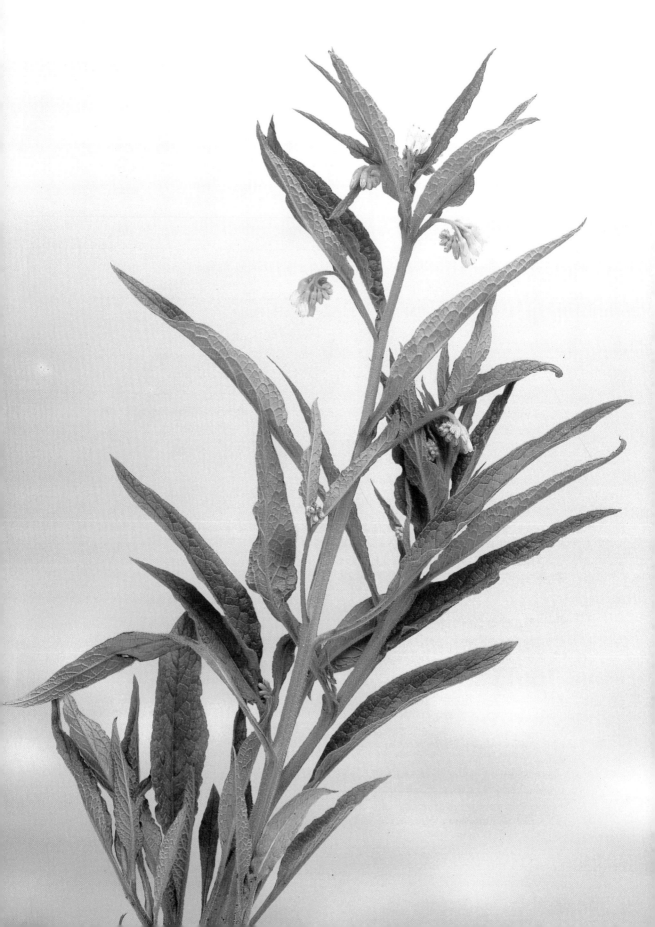

# The homeopathic remedy kit

*Many of the sixty remedies that are recommended for use in this book are essential to any home remedy kit. Others may be used once in a life time or not at all. About twenty remedies and five creams or tinctures should suffice for a basic kit but deciding exactly what to include can cause as much "agony" as that given to a music lover restricted to ten records when cast away on the fabled desert island. However the following are likely to be the most useful.*

## BASIC KIT

| Pills (6C or 30C) | | Creams/Tinctures |
|---|---|---|
| Aconite | Hypericum | Calendula (or Hypercal) |
| Apis | Ignatia | cream – for cuts and sores |
| Arnica | Ledum | Arnica cream – for bruises |
| Arsenicum | Lycopodium | Urtica (or burn |
| Belladonna | Mercurius | combination) cream |
| Bryonia | Nux vomica | Euphrasia tincture – for eyes |
| Chamomilla | Phosphorus | Rescue cream |
| Ferrum phos | Pulsatilla | |
| Gelsemium | Rhus tox | |
| Hepar sulph | Ruta | |

In addition the kit should include Rescue remedy (sometimes called First Aid Remedy) as well as bandages, plasters, tweezers, and scissors. All the items should be kept in a secure, lidded box in a cool, dry place well away from strong smells such as camphor, eucalyptus, or perfumes. Remedies should last indefinitely under these conditions. Keep the kit well out of reach of children, even though homeopathic remedies are not dangerous to small children, and it is impossible to overdose.

Add to the basic kit according to the needs of your household. For example, if you have a colicky child you may want to add Colocynth or Mag phos; Eupatorium can be good for bone-aching influenza; if piles are a problem then include Hamamelis cream and/or Aesculus cream; consider Drosera, Spongia, and Rumex if someone is always getting coughs; and if you have worked out the constitutional type of your child, then you may want to include Sulphur, Nat mur, or Calc carb.

Potency is a vexed question even for the most experienced of homeopaths. For home prescribing keep it very simple and use pills of the 6th (6C) or 30th (30C) potency. With 6C you will probably have to repeat more often.

**Where to obtain your remedies**
Health food shops and some chemists in the United Kingdom may stock the most common 6C remedies, albeit in cartons, which can be bulky to store. It is probably easiest, especially if you want to buy a number of remedies, to contact one of the major homeopathic pharmacies listed in the resources section. Most of them can supply the remedies in a useful container, will accept credit card payments or payment on delivery, and have a 24-hour answering service. Remedies are inexpensive, and the pharmacy may offer a discount if your order is large enough.

# RESOURCES

**Pharmacies**
Helios Homeopathic Pharmacy
97 Camden Road
Tunbridge Wells
Kent TN1 2QR
Tel: 0892 537254/536393

Helios are rather unique in that most of their excellent remedies are handmade.

Nelson's Pharmacy
73 Duke Street
London W1M 6BY
Tel: 071 629 3118

Ainsworths Pharmacy
38 New Cavendish Street
London W1M 7LH
Tel: 071 935 5330

**Books and Bookshops**
Books on homeopathy are legion, although most of them are for the professional and hard to find. One of the best introductions is:
*Homeopathy: Medicine of the New Man*
**George Vithoulkis** Thorsons, 1985

**Dorothy Shepherd** has written three very enjoyable general books on homeopathy all published by C W Daniel:
*Magic of the Minimum Dose*, 1964
*More Magic of the Minimum Dose*, 1974
*A Physicians Posy*, 1969

If you want to know more about the remedies you need a good Materia Medica. Two excellent ones written for the professional but in an accessible style are:
*Homeopathic Drug Pictures*
**Margaret Tyler**
C W Daniel, 1970

*Studies of Homeopathic Remedies*
**Douglas Gibson**
Beaconsfield, 1987

These books can probably be ordered through your local bookshop. Failing that try:
Watkins Bookshop
19 Cecil Court
Charing Cross Road
London WC2N 4EZ
Tel: 071 836 2182

or
Minerva Books Mail Order Service
6 Bothwell Street
London W6 8DY
Tel: 071 385 1361

**Training Courses**
Some local education authorities run evening classes in homeopathy. These can be an excellent practical introduction to the subject. If you are interested in a professional training contact one of the dozen or so colleges that are scattered throughout the country. All of them offer a four year part-time course and in some cases a three-year full-time one. For more information contact:
The Society of Homeopaths
2 Artizan Road
Northampton NN1 4HV
Tel: 0604 21400

**Finding a Homeopathic Practitioner**
As with any therapist, word of mouth recommendation is often best. If you cannot find one in your area contact The Society of Homeopaths at the address above. All practising members of the Society are graduates of one of the colleges or have passed the Society's exams. Some orthodox doctors have completed a postgraduate course in homeopathy in addition to their medical training. A few may offer homeopathy under the NHS. For more information contact:
The British Homeopathic Association
27A Devonshire Street
London W1N 1RJ
Tel: 071 935 2163

**Publisher's acknowledgements**

Gaia Books would like to thank the following for their help in the production of this book: Dr Brian Kaplan for checking the manuscript; Dr Patrick Pietroni, Joanna Godfrey Wood, Suzy Boston, and Michelle Atkinson for editorial contributions; Lesley Gilbert for text preparation; Susan Mennell for picture research, assisted by Samantha Nunn; and thanks also to Helen Spencer, Eliza Dunlop, Imogen Bright, and Gill Smith. Gaia would also like to thank the gardeners at Weleda UK Ltd for supplying a Rhus tox plant.

**Photographic credits**

**A-Z Botanical Collection** p. 47; **Heather Angel** pp. 23, 50; **Bruce Coleman** pp. 11 (Werner Stoy), 15 (Hans Reinhard), 18 (Hans Reinhard), 26 (Dr. Frieder Sauer), 31 (Hans Reinhard), 39 (Michael Fogden), 42-3 (H.J. Flugel), 55 (Hans Reinhard), 58-9 (Hans Reinhard), 78 (Jane Burton), 79 (Jane Burton); **Mary Evans Picture Library** p.8; **Gaia Books** pp. 27, 66-7, 70, 74, 83, 87, 91 (Philip Dowell); **Landscape Only** p. 6 (Joe Cornish); **Science Photo Library** pp. 2 (Gordon Garrard), 62 (A.B. Dowsett); **Wildlife Matters** p.35

# INDEX

Bold type indicates the main entries, *italic* type indicates a photograph.

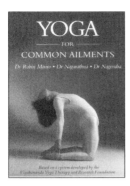

YOGA FOR
COMMON AILMENTS
Dr Nagarathna
Dr Nagendra
Dr Robin Monro
£6.99
ISBN 1 85675 010 8

Based on new research from India, this clear
and simple-to-use handbook presents a
comprehensive system of yoga therapy. It deals
with more than 35 common ailments including
stress, depression, insomnia, and heart disease,
and explains how to construct a yoga programme
tailored to treating each disease.

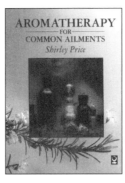

AROMATHERAPY FOR
COMMON AILMENTS
Shirley Price
£6.99
ISBN 1 85675 005 1

This is a practical self-help guide to using the
ancient system of aromatherapy for the
maintenance of good health, and for healing
common ailments. The beautiful photography
and clear, informative text provide an invaluable
reference on treating a wide range of ailments,
with advice on using home treatments.

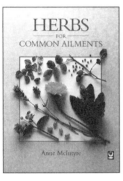

HERBS FOR
COMMON AILMENTS
Anne McIntyre
£6.99
ISBN 1 85675 055 8

An excellent introduction to this increasingly
popular natural therapy. The clear instructions
and illustrations combine with glorious full colour
photographs to show you how to identify and
prepare herbs, and how to use them simply,
effectively, and safely. A time honoured way of
relieving a whole host of everyday ailments.

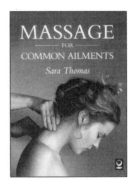

MASSAGE FOR
COMMON AILMENTS
Sara Thomas
£6.99
ISBN 1 85675 031 0

Touch is the most natural and comforting way
to heal. This book shows the basic eastern and
western massage techniques, and uses step-by-
step instructions and informative illustrations to
present clear detailed guidance on how to relieve
a whole range of everyday family health
problems. An indispensable guide.

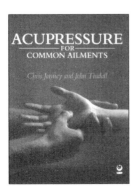

ACUPRESSURE FOR
COMMON AILMENTS
Chris Jarmey
John Tindall
£6.99
ISBN 1 85675 015 9

A self-help guide to bringing the
remarkable healing power of acupressure
to your fingertips. Simply applying pressure
to specific points on the body stimulates
subtle energy to boost the immune system
and alleviate many common ailments.

*Hypericum* This remedy can be very helpful when the bite is in a very sensitive area rich in nerves, such as the lips or finger tips. You may feel the pain shooting up the nerve tracks.

*Ledum* Use this remedy when the injury feels cold to the touch yet is better after using cold compresses. Apply the remedy as a cream or diluted tincture, or take it in pill form.

## Boils

A boil is an infected area of tissue and skin around a hair follicle. It contains a core of pus and can be extremely painful until it comes to a head and the pus discharged. Occasionally your body will absorb the boil, in which case, if there is no pain, you need no further treatment. Seek medical advice if the pain persists after a few days.

*Arsenicum*
Use Arsenicum when the boil is hot and burning yet you are able to ease the pain with hot compresses.

*Belladonna* Use this remedy in the early stages, when the boil is red and throbs violently.

*Hepar sulph* The pains are sharp and penetrating, and worse for cold. The boil is full of yellow-green pus, which may ooze out.

*Tarent cub* This remedy is very helpful when a boil develops rapidly after a slow incubation. It feels very hard, is bluish in colour and the pain is agonizing and burning.

## Bruises

A bruise forms when a blow injures the tissue under the skin without breaking it. The rupture of blood vessels makes the skin appear black and blue.

*Arnica* This is the number one remedy for bruises. Its effects often seem magical and if you use it immediately it will prevent even the most fearful blow from developing into a painful lump. Use Arnica externally or internally, or both if your bruising is severe.

*Hypericum* When the bruise is on a part of the body rich in nerves, such as fingers, toes, lips, nose, ears, or coccyx, Hypericum may be more effective than Arnica. Often you may have shooting pains from the bruising.

*Ruta* This has a special affinity with the periosteum, the membrane covering the bones, so use Ruta after a kick in the shins, or whenever the bone feels bruised.

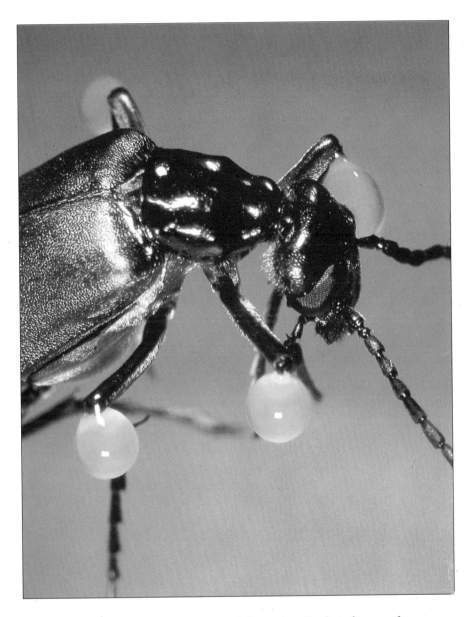

***Cantharis****, otherwise known as Spanish fly, or Blister Beetle, is the source of an excellent remedy for burning pains such as those experienced in cystitis. It is best used for acute inflammatory situations that appear suddenly.*

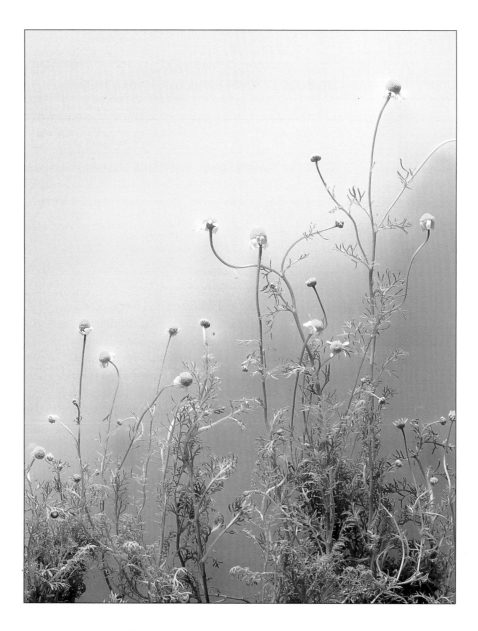

*Chamomilla* has irritability as a keynote; perfect for bad-tempered, teething babies. Older children and adults will also respond to the remedy if they are in a highly emotional, temperamental state.

## Burns

Treat minor burns or scalds, including sunburn, that sting and are painful but do not blister externally. Apply homeopathic cream of *Urtica*, *Calendula*, or *Hypercal* or tincture (diluted one part to ten parts water) immediately and liberally to the affected area. Or you can use a cream that contains a combination of these remedies. For more serious burns that begin to blister, take *Cantharis* hourly. If the burn covers an extensive area of the body (at least 5% of the surface area) seek medical help urgently. While you are waiting take *Cantharis* or *Causticum* every 15 minutes. Drink plenty as the loss of body fluids through burnt skin causes dehydration. For shock (see p. 45), alternate *Arnica* with the other remedies.

## Chickenpox

Chickenpox usually starts with a rash, which blisters and forms pustules, turning to scabs later as the pustules heal. It is a common childhood illness, that usually appears in quite a mild form in young children. Although very infectious and quite uncomfortable it is seldom serious. The disease is contagious until all the pox have turned to scabs. The same virus is also responsible for shingles, which can be extremely painful because the skin eruptions affect the nerves. Use the following chickenpox remedies for shingles, too, if the symptoms fit:

*Ant tart*  The rash is very slow to develop and the spots are full of pus. The child is very sleepy and may have a bad cough.

*Belladonna*  This remedy is most useful in the first stages of the disease. Use it when the child has a high temperature, a red face, and when the skin is hot and dry. The child may have a throbbing headache and, even if tired, may find sleeping difficult.

*Mercurius*  A useful remedy if the spots become septic. The child is sweaty and thirsty and feels worse at night.

*Pulsatilla*  This remedy is usually indicated on its emotional characteristics. The child is weepy and clingy and feels better for cool, fresh air.

*Rhus tox*  This is a particularly important remedy for chickenpox and shingles because its symptom picture (see p. 86) describes exactly the intense itching and restlessness the spots often induce. The child cannot stop scratching and may be extremely distressed because of it.

# Colds and Influenza

It can be hard to distinguish between a bad cold and mild influenza, and because names make little difference in homeopathy, both of these ailments are treated together here.

Homeopaths believe that a cold or two every year is not a bad thing, as it "cleans out" the system. There is probably little point in treating an ordinary cold – let it take its course. If you get very many colds a year then you should seek help from a professional homeopath to strengthen your immune system. Generally, if you are not beginning to feel better after a few days and you feel your body is "stuck" and needs a bit of help then consider the remedies below:

*Aconite* Use this remedy only at the beginning of the illness, and if it strikes quite suddenly, particularly at night. Exposure to cold, dry winds is often the cause of the chill. You have a fever and are rather thirsty and sweaty. You may develop a dry, painful cough.

*Allium cepa* An all-purpose cold remedy if you have a very runny nose with burning discharge. Your eyes run and smart although the resulting tears are quite bland.

*Arsenicum* The cold often starts in the nose, which produces a thin, watery, burning discharge. You sneeze a lot and the cold sometimes goes to the chest; you feel very chilly and restless but enjoy sips of water.

*Belladonna* The symptoms of high fever, red face, and burning appear very suddenly in Belladonna cases. Although your skin is dry you are not usually thirsty. Your head almost always hurts; the pain is best described as throbbing.

*Bryonia* The symptoms are slow to develop. You feel irritable and prefer to be left completely still and alone. Bryonia is a very "thirsty" remedy and you feel better for deep draughts of cold water. The remedy comes into its own after the cold has gone to your chest, producing a painful, dry cough.

*Eupatorium* This is the main remedy when the influenza has got right into your bones, which then ache. You are very thirsty and feel better for sweating, although this does not help your headache.

*Ferrum phos* A good catch-all remedy in the early stages of influenza, where there are no real prominent symptoms. You just feel generally run-down and perhaps moderately thirsty.

*Gelsemium* Shakiness and shivering are the main key notes of a Gelsemium cold or bout of influenza. Symptoms tend to develop slowly. You feel very tired and weak, and your body and muscles feel heavy. You may have a headache at the back of your head. You will only feel slight thirst, if at all.

# Colic

Colic can be a big problem to a small baby and is equally distressing to the anxious parents. It usually refers to a digestive upset with plenty of wind. The spasmodic pains are sharp and often sudden.

*Colocynthis*  The baby is very bad tempered and doubles up with pain. Applying firm pressure with the palm of your hand on the baby's tummy helps.

*Dioscorea*  The baby is not quite as angry as the Colocynthis symptoms picture, and stretches out, or tries to bend backward, to ease the pain.

*Mag phos*  The baby brings its knees up to the stomach to ease the pain. Warmth, for example from a hot water bottle, and gentle pressure help to ease the pain.

# Coughs and Croup

One cough, to the inexperienced ear, sounds very much like another. Dozens of remedies are available to cure coughs, the most common of which are given below. If these are not successful, consult a homeopathic practitioner. Croup is a dreadfully harsh-sounding cough that affects small children and keeps everyone awake at night. Try the remedies for croup given below, but seek help if you are worried or if it has persited for several days; it is sometimes dangerous.

*Aconite*  This remedy suits coughs that are hoarse, dry, and painful. They may be quite violent, which causes breathlessness, and they tend to be worse at night. Try this remedy first for croup.

*Bryonia*  These coughs are hard, dry, and painful. The chest hurts so much that you hold it while you cough. You feel worse in warm rooms and better for sitting up and taking long drinks of cold water. Bryonia can also be an excellent bronchitis remedy if the above symptoms are present.

*Drosera*  Use Drosera for an incessant barking cough. This is the kind of cough that takes your breath away; you choke to the point of retching. It feels as if a feather is tickling the inside of your throat. The cough is so deep that you may have to hold the sides of your abdomen.

*Hepar sulph*  This remedy suits painful barking coughs, which are worse for cold air or getting cold. The chest rattles and is full of mucus, which you find hard to cough up; if any does appear it will be thick and yellow. You feel weak and bad tempered. Hepar sulph is the third remedy to try for croup; use it if Aconite and Spongia fail.

*Rumex*  Every breath of fresh air causes tickling in the throat, bringing on a persistent cough. Your chest hurts and you feel better for covering your mouth. There is lots of frothy sputum.

*Spongia*  This hollow, barking cough sounds like the sawing of wood. Your chest feels full and you feel suffocated by it. Spongia is the second remedy to try for croup, if Aconite has not worked.

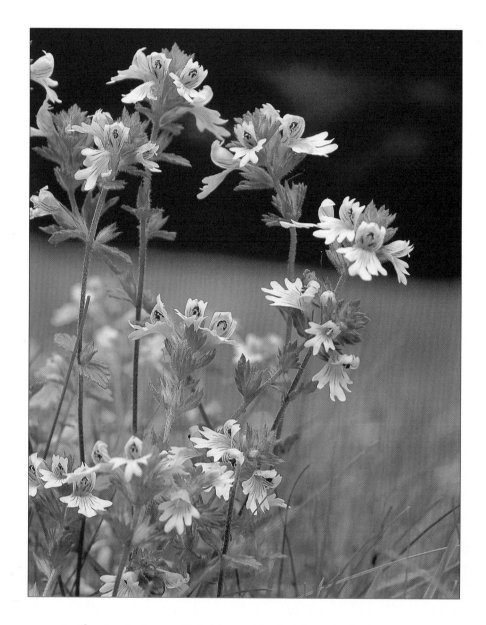

*Euphrasia*, also known as Eyebright, provides relief for tired and inflamed eyes. The remedy affects the mucous membranes, especially of the eyes. Secretions are watery and acrid.

## Cuts and Injuries

For shallow, surface wounds first clean the cut, then apply *Calendula* cream or diluted tincture. Cover with an elastoplast or a bandage if necessary. For more serious injuries, take *Calendula* in pill form as well. For deep cuts in especially sensitive places, such as finger tips or lips, use *Hypericum* or *Hypercal* cream or diluted tincture. You should dress puncture wounds, such as those caused by treading on a garden fork, with diluted *Ledum* tincture. If the wound is very deep, take *Ledum* in pill form as well.

## Cystitis

Cystitis is an acute bladder infection, particularly common in women. The symptoms are burning pains during urination and a strong desire to pass urine, but with only partial success. In persistent cases it is recommended you consult your doctor, who may want to send a urine sample away for analysis. While cystitis is less common in boys and men it can be more serious and you should seek medical help.

*Cantharis*  Try Cantharis first for cystitis. Use it when the urine is almost scalding. You will feel desperate urging with very little to show for it and the agony is extreme.

*Sarsaparilla*  This remedy covers all cystitis symptoms, but its distinguishing keynote is that the pain is worst at the close of urination.

*Causticum*  This is another remedy for burning symptoms. It can help if you experience an involuntary passage of urine on coughing in addition to the usual retention and pain.

## Diarrhoea

Diarrhoea is the body's way of quickly removing impurities and toxins from the digestive system. For this reason it is best not to interfere with such a natural process straight away. Avoid dehydration by drinking plenty of fluids. If after a day, however, it has not cleared up, try a homeopathic remedy. These remedies are useful on holiday, when food or water may easily upset the stomach.

*Arsenicum*  This remedy saves a lot of holidays. It is usually the first remedy to try for food poisoning, when the diarrhoea is often accompanied by vomiting and nausea. You will feel chilly, weak, and rather restless.

*Colocynthis*  The diarrhoea is accompanied by agonizing stomach cramps . The pain comes in waves and your intestines feel as if they are being squeezed. Doubling up eases the pain, as does hard pressure. Anger is marked – you rise to the slightest irritation.

*Phosphorus* The diarrhoea is very watery and usually painless. It will feel as if a tap has been left on. You may crave cold water, but this tends to be vomited up as soon as the stomach has warmed it through.

*Podophyllum* There are lots of gurgling sounds followed by a great torrent of painless and putrid diarrhoea. You cannot tolerate food or drink.

*Veratrum alb* This is a real emergency remedy. Not only do you have diarrhoea, but violent vomiting as well. The symptoms also include profuse sweating, coldness, and painful cramps that may even lead to collapse. You will crave ice-cold water.

## Earache

The ear is a complex organ and an earache may be one of several kinds. An infection of the middle ear, otitis media, is the most common cause and can be persistent in children. Orthodox medicine usually treats it with antibiotics if a bacterial cause is suspected. The pain may be accompanied by fever and deafness. Always seek medical advice if the pain persists or is intolerable, as the eardrum may be on the point of rupturing. Homeopathy can be helpful in both acute cases and in the chronic condition. If the ailment keeps recurring, however, take the child to a qualified homeopath. Check first to see if there is a foreign body lodged in the ear. You may need help from a doctor with this.

*Aconite* Sudden onset is always a keynote of Aconite conditions. The symptoms are often brought on after being out in the cold. The child will appear very fearful; the worst time is around midnight and for about two hours after.

*Belladonna* Symptoms come on very quickly. The earache is intensely painful; the ear throbs and looks red. The temperature may be high.

*Chamomilla* The pain can be excruciating and the child responds by becoming extremely bad tempered. You may be able to ameliorate this by carrying or rocking the child. Warmth helps to ease the pain.

*Ferrum phos* The pain comes on gradually and the remedy is best used in the early stages. Use it if Belladonna has not worked.

*Hepar sulph* This remedy works better in the middle stages of inflammation, when pus is beginning to build up. The child may have a sore throat and a cold with thick yellow-green discharge. The pain is sharp and the child will feel cross and needs warmth.

*Mercurius* The pain may extend to the throat and mouth, sometimes with a nasal discharge that is yellow and occasionally blood-streaked. The glands in the face and neck may be swollen and hard. The child is likely to be thirsty and sweaty, and have lots of saliva that smells bad.

*Pulsatilla* The aches may come and go with no pattern to them. The child is weepy and irritable, but better for affection and sympathy. The child feels more comfortable if the room is kept cool.

*Verbascum (Mullein oil)* This is a very helpful and soothing external application. You can use it in addition to other remedies, or by itself. Apply a few warmed drops into the affected ear.

## Eye Injuries

Try *Arnica* first for injuries with bruising. If this is insufficient, and the eye becomes cold and bloodshot, use *Ledum* internally and externally. The remedy *Symphytum* has a special affinity with the eyeball. Consider it when the eye has taken the full force of a hard object, such as a tennis ball.

## Eye Strain

The frequent use of the modern VDU has probably overtaken reading and writing in bad light as the main source of eye strain. Ensure that you rest your eyes regularly when using one over a long period of time.

*Euphrasia*  This is the traditional remedy for tired eyes that water and burn. It is easiest to use externally in diluted tincture form.

*Ruta*  This is another good remedy for sore eyes. Ruta can be very useful after too much close work has made your vision dim.

## Eyes – Inflammation

Remedies are included here for conjunctivitis and blepharitis. Conjunctivitis is an inflammation of the mucous membrane that covers and protects the front of the eye, and which also lines the lids. Blepharitis is an inflammation of the eyelids themselves.

Eyes are the most delicate of organs; seek medical advice if you are worried or if an inflammation has not cleared up after a few days of treatment. Bathe the eyes frequently and wash your hands immediately afterwards to prevent the infection spreading.

*Aconite*  Your eyes feel hot and dry, as if a piece of grit is in them. They look red and inflamed and the eyelids are swollen. The symptoms are often caused by being out in a cold wind or being caught in a draught.

*Apis*  This remedy is especially good when your eyelids are red and puffy and are filled with fluid. You can use it when your eyeballs appear red and swollen, and burn. Cold compresses ease the discomfort considerably.

*Belladonna*  Your eyes burn, feel dry, and look bloodshot. The pupils are dilated. You are very sensitive to light and prefer to be in a darkened room. The symptoms appear quickly.

*Euphrasia*  This is best used externally as a diluted tincture. Put a few drops into a small container of sterilized water. Your eyes burn and water profusely; the lids may feel rather sticky.

*Pulsatilla*  Eye ailments that need Pulsatilla are characterized by a yellow discharge that is quite bland – it does not burn or irritate. Your eyes and lids are sore and swollen and the lids might be sticky as well.

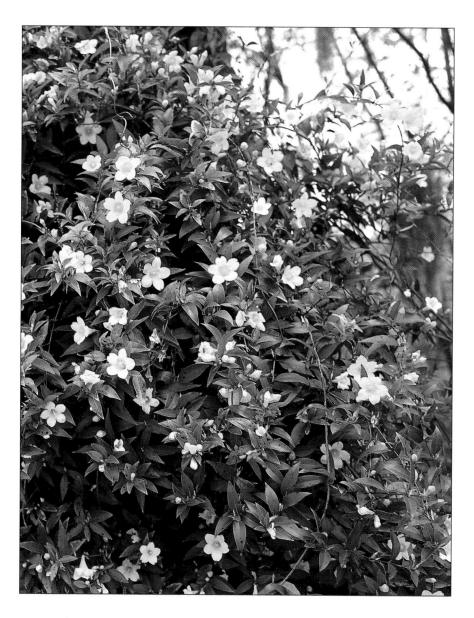

***Gelsemium***, *a North American plant, is the source of a major remedy for 'flu and anxious states. The remedy profoundly affects the muscles and motor nerves resulting in weakness, trembling, and heaviness.*

## Eyes – Styes

A stye is a small boil on the eyelid. It may look quite alarming if the eye closes up, but homeopathic treatment usually brings a response. In addition to the remedies listed below, consider also those included under Boils and Eye Inflammation (see pp. 25 and 34).

*Pulsatilla*  Use this remedy for styes, especially those that recur and discharge yellow pus. These styes are more common on the upper lids.

*Staphysagria*  These styes may follow a period of emotional stress; notably after unexpressed anger has been bottled up.

## Fainting and Collapse

The symptoms of fainting are coldness, paleness, and dizziness, and in severe cases complete loss of consciousness brought on by a drop in the supply of blood to the brain. The causes are varied; they include shock, severe pain, extreme tiredness or hunger, emotional shock, and very occasionally, something more serious. Usually the sufferer will feel better after 10 to 15 minutes. If not, and there is no obvious reason for fainting, seek medical help immediately. Ensure that the person's head is not higher than the body, but otherwise do not move the person until he or she feels ready to. Then give a glass of water with the Rescue Remedy in it (see p. 90). If the person is unconscious, moisten the lips with Rescue Remedy continuously every few minutes. If the cause is shock keep the person warm. If the person is doing well after about 15 minutes you may not need to give a remedy. Otherwise consider the following treatments:

*Aconite*  Use Aconite for sudden shock resulting from intense fright and anxiety. The person feels that s/he is going to die, and the fear lingers on after the sufferer has seemingly recovered.

*Arnica*  This is usually the first remedy to use for shock that follows an accident involving physical pain or injury.

*Carbo veg*  Nicknamed the "corpse reviver", it is used when the person looks cold and still and is very slow to come round. It is a good remedy for collapse from exhaustion.

*China*  Use this remedy for fainting and weakness caused by loss of fluids, whether from vomiting, diarrhoea, or loss of blood.

*Ignatia*  This acts on the emotions and you should give it when fainting occurs on hearing bad news or of an emotional loss.

*Pulsatilla*  Give Pulsatilla when a warm and stuffy atmosphere is the cause of fainting. A very "emotional" remedy, if you know the person use it if they are gentle, mild mannered, and give up easily.

**Food Poisoning** – see Diarrhoea (p.32) or Nausea and Vomiting (p.44)

# Fractures

Homeopathy can speed up the healing time for broken bones once the fracture has received medical attention and been properly set. However, at the time of the break, as with any accident, it is a good idea to take *Arnica* for the bruising and shock.

*Calc phos* Calcium and phosphorus are the two main minerals needed for building up healthy bones. Use Calc phos after the bone has properly knitted (see Symphytum, right) and give it daily until fully healed. It is also a good remedy for people with weak or brittle bones that are prone to fractures.

*Symphytum* Give Symphytum, also called Knitbone, daily for a month or two after setting, until the bone has knitted together.

# Grief

In homeopathy emotional symptoms are considered every bit as important as physical ones, and in chronic disease they are usually treated with even more importance. Unresolved emotional issues, such as grief, can get "locked up" in the body and cause physical havoc later when they surface in another guise. Although homeopathy cannot "cure" grief – there has to be a natural period of mourning – it can ease the process. Serious problems arising from deep grief are best dealt with by a professional homeopath, but here are two remedies that can often help:

*Ignatia* This is usually the first remedy to try in the initial stages of grief, especially if you are in a highly weepy, emotional, and oversensitive state, perhaps even hysterical at times. Sighing is a big Ignatia keynote. Ignatia is very suitable after all kinds of grief, including the end of a relationship or after a bereavement.

*Nat mur* Always try this if Ignatia does not act or fails to hold. You will be tearful and emotional, but the grief is less open and you prefer to cry alone in the privacy of you own room. Conversely, you may be so deeply affected that you cannot cry at all. Consolation may make things worse. Nat mur can be suitable for more long-term sadness, when you feel you should be getting over it but have got "stuck".

# Haemorrhoids (piles)

Haemorrhoids are varicose veins around the anal canal. They often protrude or rupture and can be extremely painful. Blood discharged while passing stools is a symptom. Fortunately homeopathy can help and remedies can be used both internally and externally. If the following do not help the ailment may be deep seated, and you need constitutional treatment.

*Aesculus*　For burning piles (possibly extruding and resembling a bunch of purple grapes), accompanied by sharp, shooting pains up your back, apply Aesculus cream.

*Hamamelis*　The piles are very bruised and sore, with a bursting feeling and they continually bleed. Use Hamamelis as a cream. (Use it also to soothe the pain of varicose veins in the legs.)

# Hayfever

Hayfever is very much a 20th-century disease. It was much less common 100 years ago, even though far more people then lived on farms close to the grasses and pollens that trigger off the well-known irritation. Hayfever is an allergy affecting the nose and eyes; its cause is a weakened immune system. It can be an extremely stubborn ailment to treat since a permanent cure depends on raising the quality of the immune system. A professional homeopath can do this through constitutional treatment; even so, it may take two or three seasons to eradicate the problem completely. The remedies included here will lessen the discomfort, but they will not effect a permanent cure.

*Allium cepa*　This remedy is made from the red onion, so most of us have experienced its symptoms. They include a streaming nose with a burning discharge, and watery, stinging eyes with bland secretions. You may experience violent sneezing and a tickling cough.

*Euphrasia*　This remedy has a special affinity with the eyes, so it is most suitable when your eyes cause you the biggest problem. The symptoms of Euphrasia are the converse of Allium cepa; the tears burn, but the secretions from the nose are bland.

*Arsenicum*　Use Arsenicum when the mucous membranes of the eyes and nose are affected and the secretions are extremely acrid. The nose produces a thin, watery discharge, but can also feel stuffed up, a similar feeling to the onset of a cold. You sneeze without relief.

*Sabadilla*　Use Sabadilla to ease continuous and violent sneezing and frustrating itching and tickling in the nose. One nostril may be blocked up while the other streams perhaps worsened by the smell of flowers. Your eyes also water and burn.

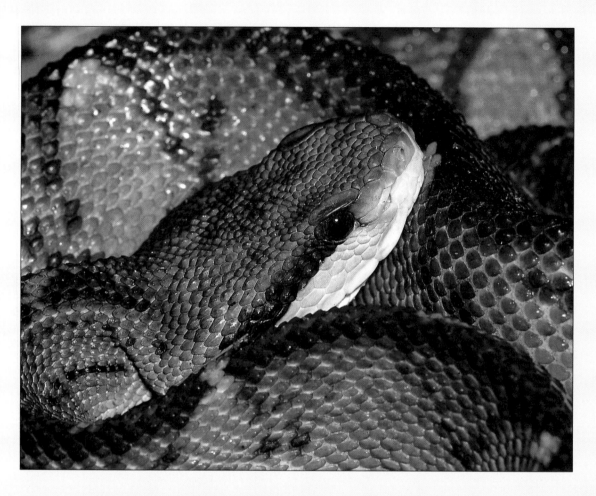

***Lachesis.*** *The venom of the South American Bushmaster snake is the most important of the snake remedies used in homeopathy. Once the poison has been potentized (see p.12), all the harm has been removed and the remedy is safe to use.*

## Indigestion

Overeating and drinking place a strain on the digestive system and are a major cause of the discomfort of indigestion. Symptoms are heartburn, wind, cramping, hiccoughs, and sometimes nausea. The problem will often ease itself without a remedy. However, for emergencies you can try the following two remedies:

*Lycopodium*  Many Lycopodium types have a fundamental weakness in the digestive system and a tendency toward anxiety. You may have a sweet tooth and eating just a little can create a sensation of fullness. Often heartburn – a feeling of burning rising from the stomach – can be a problem. Wind and muscle cramps are common. Avoid eating beans and cabbages, which cause flatulence.

*Nux vomica*  The typical Nux vomica type loves good food and drink and is rather prone to over-indulging. The food lies like a great load in your stomach, resulting in hiccoughs, heartburn, and nausea. You know that if only you could vomit, you would feel better, but somehow this is not possible. Nux vomica is also known as a good hangover remedy.

## Influenza - see Colds and Influenza (p.29)

## Measles

Measles is a particularly infectious viral disease, mainly affecting young children. The diagnosis can often be confirmed in the early stages by the appearance of small white spots within the mouth on the inside of the cheeks. The main symptoms are fever, nasal discharge, and a nasty cough followed by a rash starting on the face and spreading in great blotches all over the body. The sufferer has an aversion to light. Once the rash has finished developing, the temperature drops and the child starts to feel better.

Measles has a long incubation period and is very contagious both before and after the rash. It is not normally a dangerous disease to a healthy, well-nourished child, but you should seek medical advice as there can be rare complications.

*Aconite*  This is an excellent remedy to give in the first stages, before the rash has started and even before you are sure that it is measles. Use it if fever, croupy cough, watery nose, red eyes, and restlessness appear very suddenly.

*Apis*  The child is extremely restless with the fever, but has no thirst despite the burning heat. The eyes are inflamed and look red and puffy. Drowsiness will be noticeable, but the child has difficulty in getting to sleep.

*Belladonna*  Like Aconite, use Belladonna in the early stages of measles. The child has a very red face with high fever, but no thirst. The pupils appear enlarged and the child cannot bear the light.

*Bryonia*  It is important that the rash develops fully in measles. Use Bryonia if the rash appears very slowly or does not come up properly. There is a dry and painful chesty cough; the child wants to be left absolutely still, as movement aggravates the chest and the aching muscles. The child's mouth is very dry and wants long drinks of cold water.

*Gelsemium*  Gelsemium cases develop very slowly. The child feels very tired and weak, the eyelids feel heavy and the back of the head may ache. The symptoms feel rather like influenza, with shivering, lassitude, and aching muscles. The child will feel hot and cold by turns and will not be thirsty.

*Pulsatilla*  This remedy comes into its own once the rash has developed. There may be thick yellow mucus and sticky eyelids. The child will suffer from a slight fever, is not thirsty, and feels better in a cool room. The cough is dry at night and loose during the day.

## Mumps

Mumps is an infectious viral disease that mainly affects children. Fever accompanies a swelling of the salivary glands, especially the parotids, situated under and in the front of the ear lobes. The swelling can last four to ten days, during which time eating and drinking sour substances can be painful. It is usually a mild disease, but seek medical advice as a swelling of the parotid gland may be due to a calculus and require surgery.

*Aconite*  This is a good remedy to use when symptoms appear very suddenly. The child appears anxious, restless, and thirsty.

*Apis*  The swollen glands look particularly puffy, flushed, and feel very tender. The child is restless and hot, and wants to be kept cool, but will not usually be thirsty.

*Belladonna*  All Belladonna cases are characterized by the sudden onset of a high temperature and a red, throbbing face. The glands are very swollen and painful, especially on the right side.

*Bryonia*  The glands come up very slowly and feel hard, tender, and painful. Irritability and marked thirst are keynotes. The child wants to remain still because the slightest movement hurts.

*Mercurius*  This remedy has a strong affinity with the glands, which makes it particularly helpful in mumps. There is profuse saliva and thirst, and the breath smells bad. The child is sweaty, cross, and is alternately hot and cold.

*Pulsatilla*  The characteristic Pulsatilla emotional symptoms of weepiness and dependency are present, as well as a general lack of thirst and the need for cool air. Pulsatilla is strongly indicated if the swelling moves to the testicles or breasts.

*Rhus tox*  People who need Rhus tox always exhibit extreme restlessness. The left side of the face may be the most swollen, or the swelling may have started on the left side. Like Pulsatilla, Rhus tox can help if the testicles are swollen. The child feels better for being kept warm.

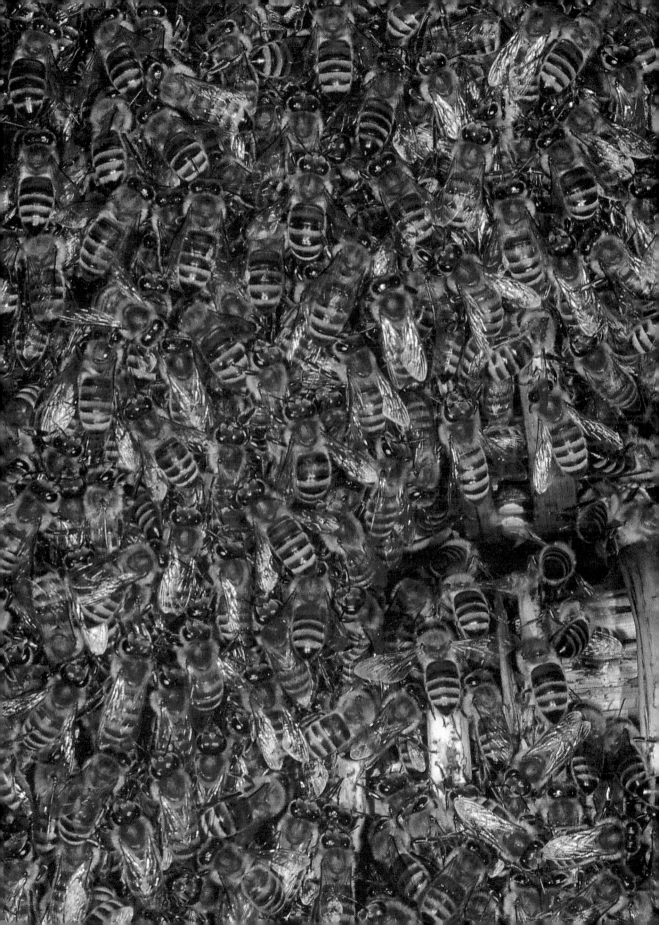